DOUBLE END BAG WORKOUT

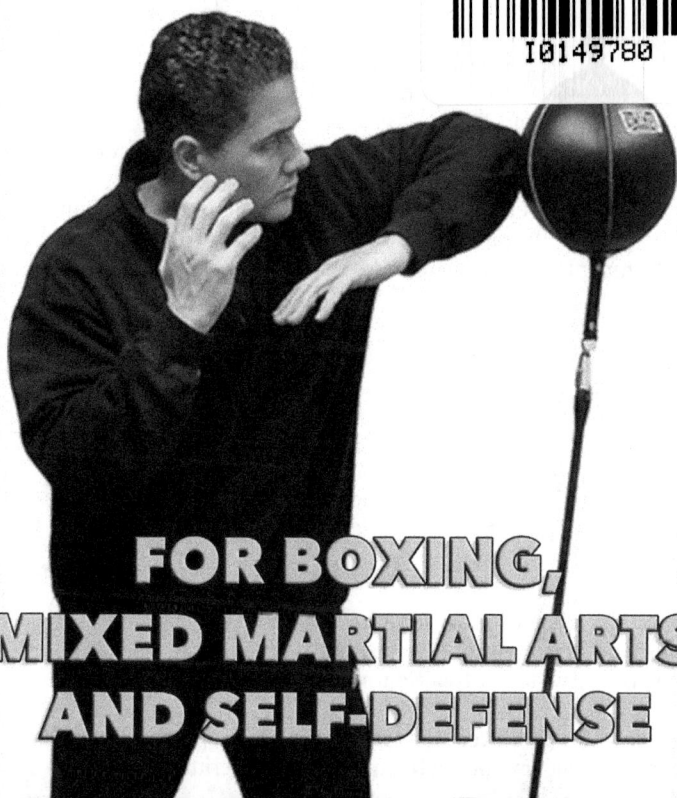

FOR BOXING, MIXED MARTIAL ARTS AND SELF-DEFENSE

SAMMY FRANCO

Also by Sammy Franco

The Heavy Bag Bible
The Widow Maker Compendium
Invincible: Mental Toughness Techniques for Peak Performance
Bruce Lee's 5 Methods of Attack
Unleash Hell: A Step-by-Step Guide to Devastating Widow Maker Combinations
Feral Fighting: Advanced Widow Maker Fighting Techniques
The Widow Maker Program: Extreme Self-Defense for Deadly Force Situations
Savage Street Fighting: Tactical Savagery as a Last Resort
Heavy Bag Workout
Heavy Bag Combinations
Heavy Bag Training
The Complete Body Opponent Bag Book
Stand and Deliver: A Street Warrior's Guide to Tactical Combat Stances
Maximum Damage: Hidden Secrets Behind Brutal Fighting Combinations
First Strike: End a Fight in Ten Seconds or Less!
The Bigger They Are, The Harder They Fall
Self-Defense Tips and Tricks
Kubotan Power: Quick & Simple Steps to Mastering the Kubotan Keychain
Gun Safety: For Home Defense and Concealed Carry
Out of the Cage: A Guide to Beating a Mixed Martial Artist on the Street
Warrior Wisdom: Inspiring Ideas from the World's Greatest Warriors
War Machine: How to Transform Yourself Into a Vicious and Deadly Street Fighter
1001 Street Fighting Secrets
When Seconds Count: Self-Defense for the Real World
Killer Instinct: Unarmed Combat for Street Survival
Street Lethal: Unarmed Urban Combat

Double End Bag Workout

ISBN: 978-1-941845-25-7
Printed in the United States of America

Published by Contemporary Fighting Arts, LLC.
Visit us Online at: **SammyFranco.com**
Follow us on Twitter: **@RealSammyFranco**

For author interviews or publicity information, please send inquiries in care of the publisher.

Contents

"To become a champion, fight one more round."

– James Corbett

Caution!

The author, publisher, and distributors of this book disclaim any liability from loss, injury, or damage, personal or otherwise, resulting from the information and procedures in this book. This book is for academic study only.

The information contained in this book is not designed to diagnose, treat, or manage any physical health conditions.

Before you begin any exercise or activity, including those suggested in this book, it is important to check with your physician to see if you have any condition that might be aggravated by strenuous training.

About this book

Double End Bag Workout is a comprehensive book written for anyone who wants to learn how to use and ultimately master the double end bag. Practitioners who use this text as a reference tool will establish a rock solid foundation for double end bag training. In fact, the skills and techniques featured in this book will significantly improve your fighting skills, enhance your conditioning, and introduce you to new aspects of working out on the bag.

The skills and techniques featured in this book will also help you achieve maximum training performance in a variety of recreational activities and professions, including boxing, mixed martial arts, martial arts (traditional and eclectic) kickboxing, self-defense, and personal fitness.

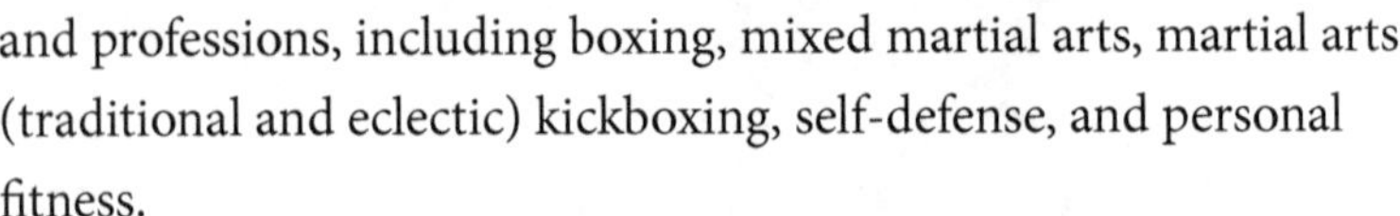

This comprehensive book covers a broad range of double end bag skills that will allow to maximize your workouts. In this information-packed guide, you'll find answers to the most important questions about double end bag training.

You will also find a section devoted to punching combinations, designed for the beginner, intermediate and advanced practitioner.

Finally, I have included several ***out of the box*** workout routines that will maximize your fighting skills for boxing, mixed martial arts, kickboxing, self-defense, and personal fitness. It features beginner, intermediate, and advanced workout routines that will improve your hand speed, timing, attack rhythm, accuracy, punching combinations, defense skills, footwork, and endurance.

All of information and knowledge featured in this book are based on my 30+ years of research, training and teaching the martial arts, boxing, and related disciplines. In fact, I have taught these unique skills to thousands of my students, and I'm confident they will help you reach higher levels of training performance.

Double End Bag Workout has six chapters, each one covers a critical aspect of training. In addition, you will also find a glossary of terms at the end of the book. Since this is both a skill-building workbook and training guide, feel free to write in the margins, underline passages, and dog-ear the pages.

Finally, I encourage you to read this book from beginning to end, chapter by chapter. Only after you have read the entire book should you treat it as a reference and skip around, reading those chapters that directly apply to you.

Train hard!

- ***Sammy Franco***

Chapter 1
The Double End Bag

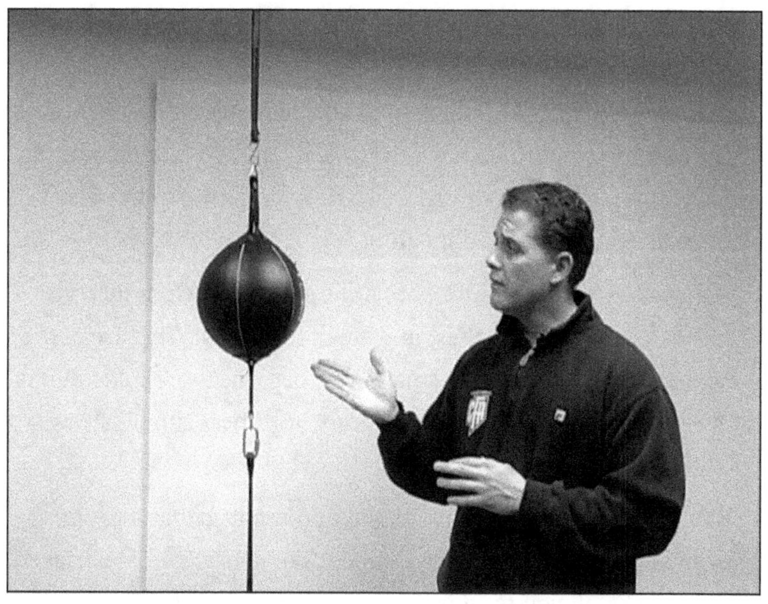

Double End Bag Characteristics

The double end bag is a unique piece of workout equipment used by boxers, kick boxers, martial artists, self-defense practitioners, as well as fitness enthusiasts. Depending on where you train and who you talk to, the double end bag is also called a top and bottom bag, floor to ceiling ball, crazy bag, headache bag, and reflex bag.

Double end bags are small, inflatable lightweight round bags that are most often constructed of vinyl or leather. This unique training bag is suspended in the air using two durable elastic cables that anchor it to the ceiling and the floor.

They also come in a variety of different sizes including large (9 inches), medium (7 inches) and small (6 inches). The size of the double end bag matters. The smaller the bag, the more difficult it is to hit it when training. As a rule of thumb, beginners should always start off with a large size bag.

Double end bags also have slightly different shape variations. They include the standard bag, double-double bag, and Mexican style bag. However, all you need is the standard version of the bag.

Double end bags are used to develop specific fighting attributes required for boxing, martial arts, and self-defense. These attributes include hand speed, timing, attack rhythm, accuracy, combination skills, defensive techniques, footwork, and endurance. Double end bags, however, are not designed for power punching.

Be forewarned! The double end bag requires a considerable amount of practice and a hell of a lot of patience. In fact, it's probably one of the most difficult pieces of boxing equipment to master.

For example, when you strike on the bag, it immediately reacts by swinging right back at you. In fact, the harder you hit the bag, the faster is rebounds. Therefore, to properly control the movement of the bag, you must strike it directly in the center. If you don't hit it dead center, it will bounce uncontrollably to the right or left.

Since double end bag training is a popular form of working out, you can find just about every type of bag variation by surfing the Internet. However, be prepared, it can be a bit overwhelming as there are so many on the market.

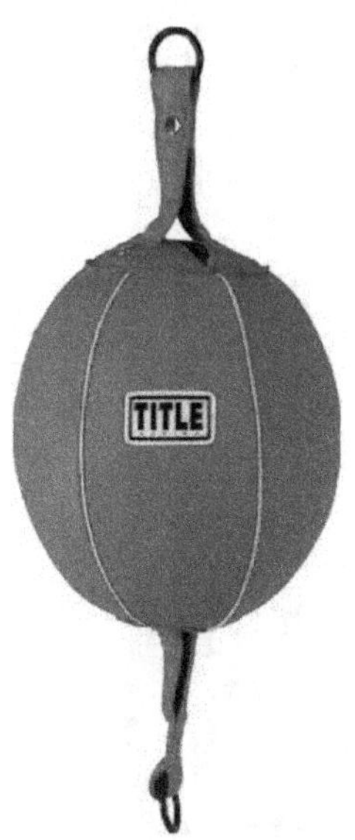

The standard double end bag.

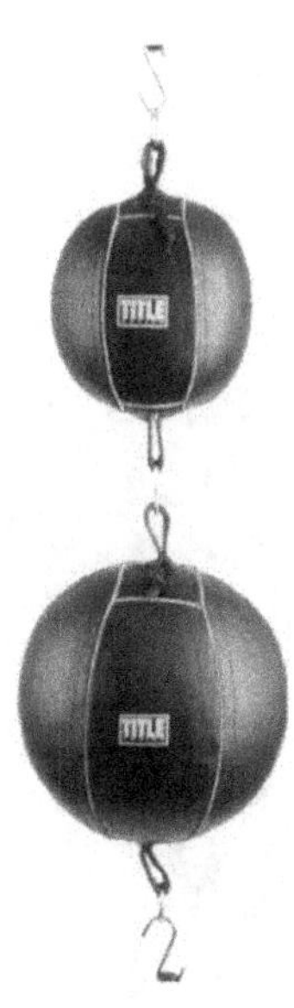

The double-double end bag.

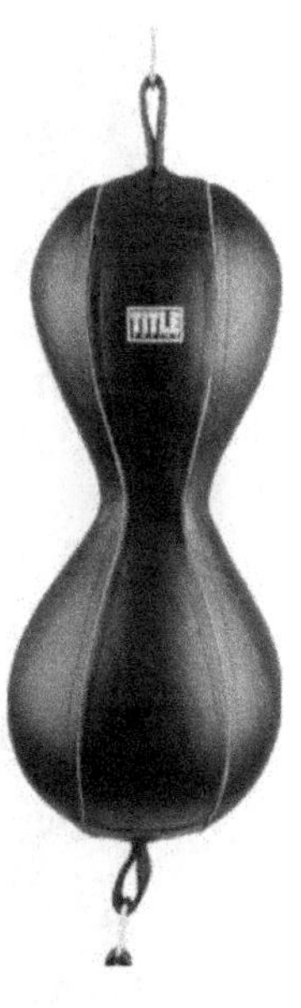

The Mexican style double end bag.

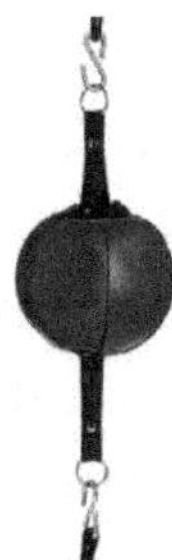

The double-double end bag can be used for developing both head and body punches.

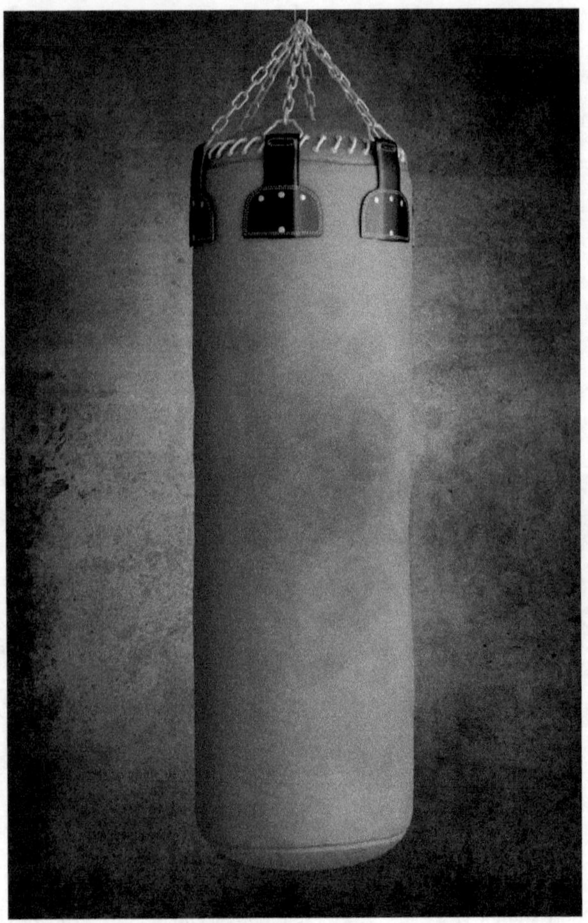

The double end bag isn't designed for punching power. If power punching is your goal, the heavy bag would be a much better alternative.

Buying a Double End Bag

When looking to buy a double end bag, avoid purchasing it from your local sporting goods store, as most of these bags are cheap, poorly made, and won't provide years of reliable use. The double end bag is a serious piece of training equipment, so you should spare no expense and look for the highest quality brand that you can afford. Not only will it provide years of reliable use, but it will help ensure a better workout.

Again, you can find a reasonably priced quality bag on the Internet. Here are just a few reputable companies:

- **Ringside Equipment (ringside.com)**
- **Combat Sports, Inc (combatsports.com)**
- **Title Boxing (titleboxing.com)**
- **Tuf-Wear (tufweardirect.com)**

Benefits of Double End Bag Training

The double end bag is a fantastic piece of training equipment that also provides a full range of benefits for the practitioner. In this section, I'm going to discuss some of the many benefits that come from regularly working out on the bag.

Cardiovascular Conditioning

If you workout on the double end bag with a significant amount of intensity, you can turn it into a challenging cardiovascular workout. However, this will require you to push yourself and throw your punches at a very respectable pace. Keep in mind, if you deliver your blows maximum speed and intensity, your workout will quickly become an anaerobic workout, and you'll most likely fizzle out.

Double end bag sessions can last anywhere from 30 seconds to 5 minutes depending on your level of conditioning, personal goals and training objectives. Much more is discussed in Chapter 6.

Improving Muscle Tone

Double end bag training can also improve the muscle tone in your entire body including your back, chest, shoulders, arms, chest, abdominals, legs, and calves. A typical workout can also burn a significant amount of calories and, therefore, can be a useful method for stripping fat from your body.

While double end bag training does improve muscle tone, it should not be used as a substitute for weight training. For those of you who want to achieve noticeable strength gains, I strongly encourage a progressive resistance exercise program.

Developing Fighting Technique

The double end bag is also a fantastic piece of equipment for developing your fighting skills and techniques. It is no surprise that boxers, kickboxers, self-defense practitioners, MMA fighters, and martial artists of all styles and backgrounds regularly use the double end bag for developing their particular style of fighting.

As you can imagine, a wide variety of punches and strikes can be developed and ultimately perfected on the bag. Some techniques include:

- *Jab*
- *Lead straight punch*
- *Rear cross*
- *Hook punches*
- *Shovel hooks*
- *Uppercut*
- *Elbow strikes*
- *Head Butt*
- *Palm heels*
- *Finger jabs*
- *Hammer fists*

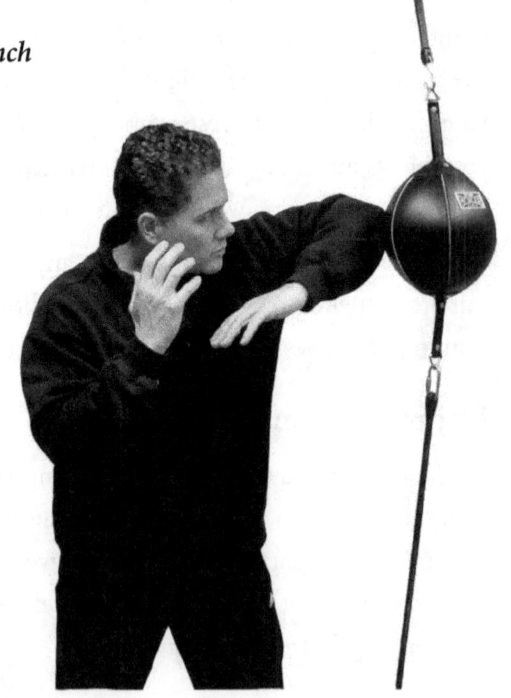

Developing Fighting Attributes

Fighting attributes are unique qualities that enhance or amplify a particular fighting skill or technique. They might include speed, power, timing, agility, ambidexterity, coordination, combat conditioning as well as many others.

The double end bag is an ideal piece of equipment for developing some of these fighting attributes. They include:

- *Punching speed*
- *Attack rhythm*
- *Ambidexterity*
- *Offensive timing*
- *Defensive timing*
- *Defensive skills*
- *Compound attack skills*
- *Balance*
- *Eye/Hand coordination*
- *Footwork skills*
- *Non-telegraphic movement*
- *Muscular relaxation*
- *Distancing*
- *Striking accuracy*

Effective Stress Reduction Tool

There's no escaping the fact that mental stress can do a tremendous amount of damage by causing heart disease, high blood pressure, chest pain and an irregular heartbeat. It's no wonder stress is called the silent killer.

The good news is, working out on the double end bag on a regular basis can be an excellent form of stress reduction. Punching and kicking an inanimate object, such as a double end bag, permits you to channel pent-up aggression in a productive fashion.

Anger Management Tool

Unless you live on your own island, you will most likely live in a populated region that puts you in contact with many people every day. Add a hectic lifestyle to the mix and you will probably encounter occasional conflicts with difficult and belligerent people.

In such situations, you will sometimes get a sudden urge to respond in a physical manner, but as a law-abiding citizen, you must repress these primitive urges. Working out on the double end bag allows you to vent toxic anger in an acceptable and appropriate way.

Inexpensive Investment

Finally, for the people on a tight budget, the good news is that double end bag training is inexpensive. Essentially, all you need is a quality bag and a good pair of gloves to protect your hands. Please see Chapter 2 to learn more about essential training gear.

Chapter 2
Getting Started

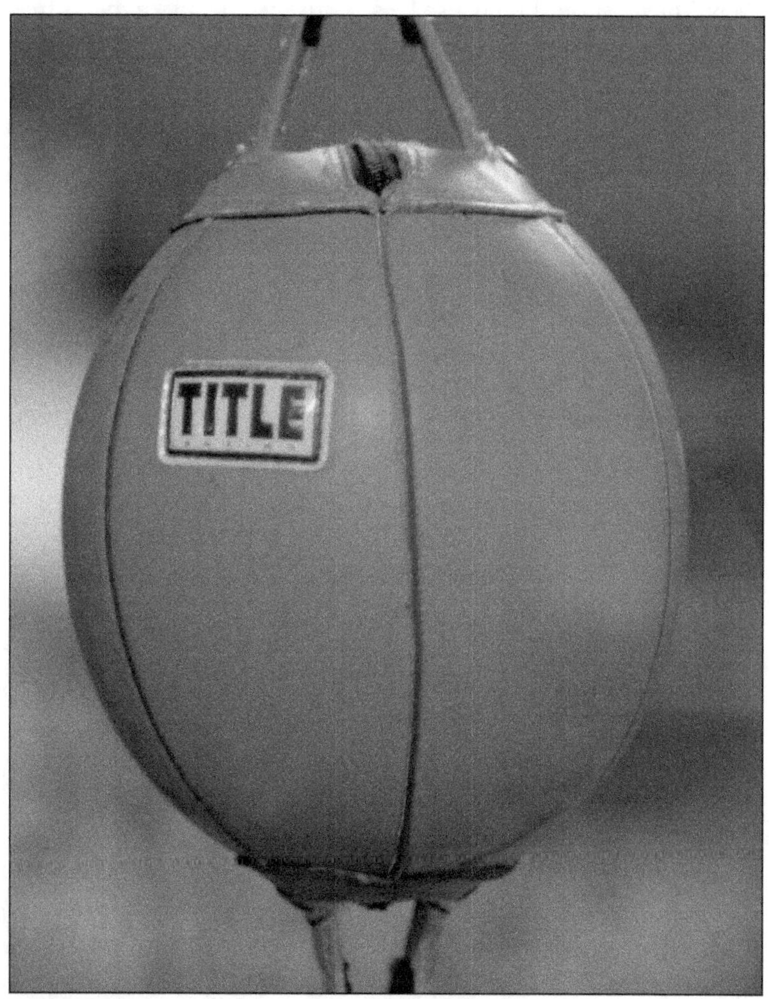

Finding the Right Place to Train

One of the most important considerations when setting up the double end bag is finding the right location for working out. First, you will need a place that will allow both you and the bag to move around freely. The location should also be a relatively quiet place that is free of distractions. Here are a few places you might want to consider when setting up your bag:

- *Garage*
- *Carport*
- *Basement*
- *Barn*
- *Home gym (if you're fortunate enough)*
- *Open field or backyard*
- *Warehouse*
- *Under a deck*

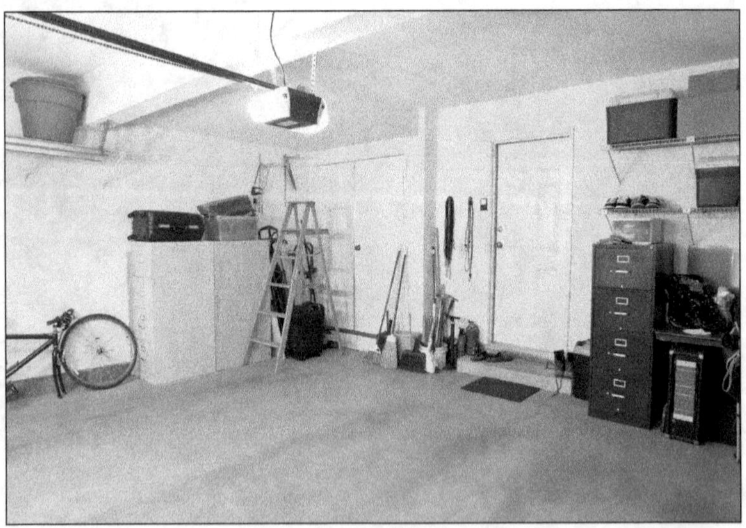

If you can manage to clear out the clutter from your garage, it can be a perfect place for working out on the bag.

Hanging the Double End Bag

Once you have found a suitable location to set up the bag, your next task is to hang it up. While there are many different ways to hang the double end bag, the most important criterion is to attach the bag to a stable structure that will allow you to suspend the ball to both the ceiling and the floor.

Most double end bags will come with two equal length elastic rubber cables or bungee straps that allow you to anchor it to the ceiling and the floor. To attach the bungee straps to the bag, simply hook each one to the metal ring sewn into each end of the bag. Then join the top elastic cable to the ceiling and the bottom one to the floor.

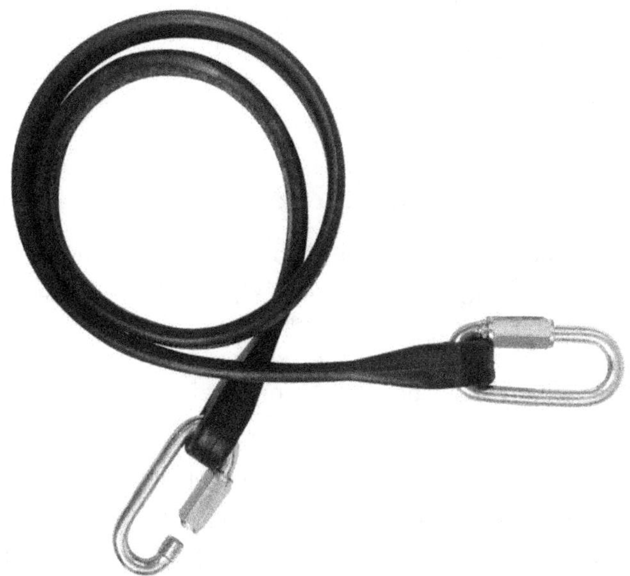

Pictured here, heavy-duty rubber straps with caribiners at both ends.

Double End Bag Hangers

Most people will be able to hang their double end bag from either a wood or steel beam located in either their basement or garage. Luckily, there are several commercial hangers that will allow you to quickly and easily hang your bag. If, however, it's not possible to hang your bag from a beam, there are wall mount hangers that can be bolted into the wall studs.

Different Types of Double End Bag Hangers

- *Steel I-Beam hanger*
- *Rafter hanger*
- *Wood Beam T-Swivel hanger*
- *Flat Wood Beam hanger*
- *Wall Mount hanger*

Double End Bag Anchors

Once the bag is suspended to the ceiling, you'll need to secure the bottom strap to the floor with an anchor. There are two types: bolt down and disc anchors.

The bolt down anchor is a D-ring that is literally bolted or screwed the into the floor. The disc anchor (sometimes called a rock anchor) is a heavy-duty disc shaped PVC bladder that is filled with either water or sand. When filled to capacity, the disc anchor weighs anywhere from 45 to 70 pounds and provides excellent stability. Most people prefer using the bag anchor because it's portable, and allows you to secure the double bag without having to drill holes in the floor.

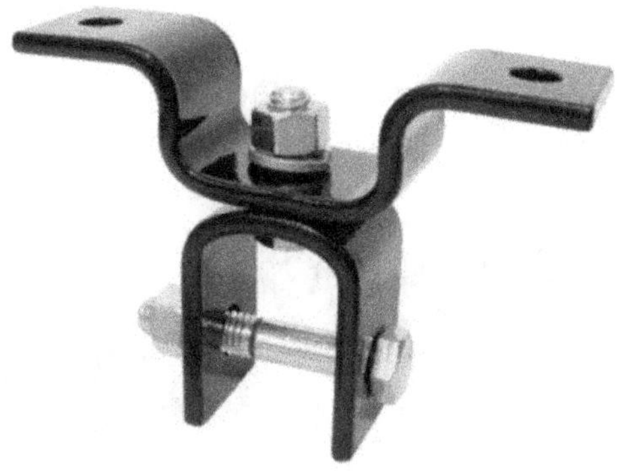

Pictured here, a wood beam double end bag hanger.

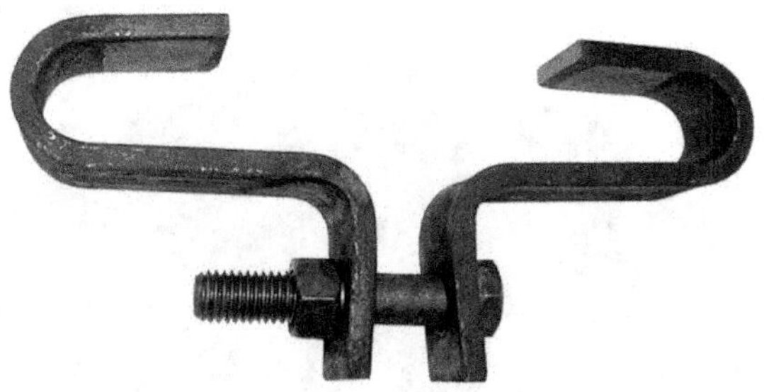

Pictured here, a steel I-beam double end bag hanger.

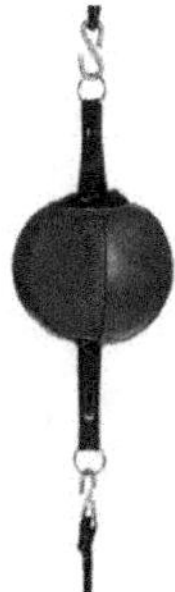

Double end bag training outdoors is a great experience. However, exposing your bag to the elements, for a prolonged period, will quickly destroy your bag. Be sure to bring your bag indoors at the end of every workout.

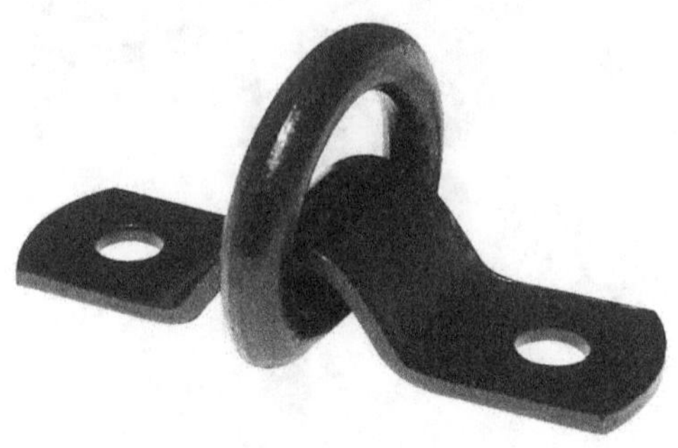

Pictured here, a bolt down floor anchor.

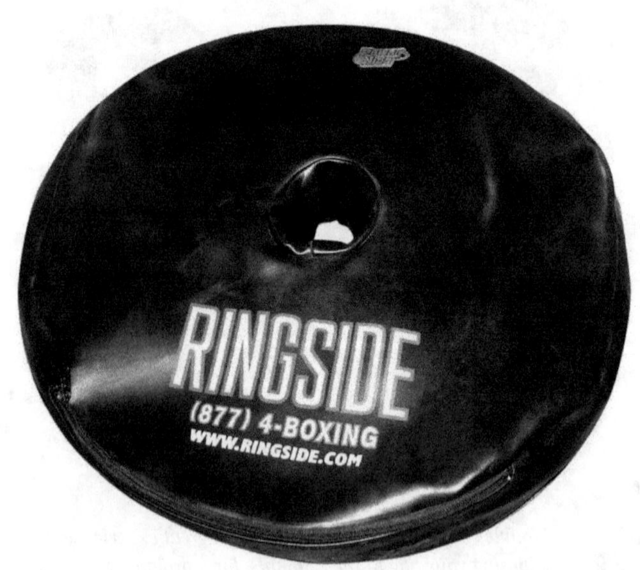

A disc anchor.

The Bag Stand

Finally, if you do not have access to a solid beam or a wall stud but do have the space, you might want to consider investing in a bag stand. These free-standing units can be used for both the heavy bag and double end bag. The only real drawback to using a stand is they limit your ability to move 360 degrees around the bag.

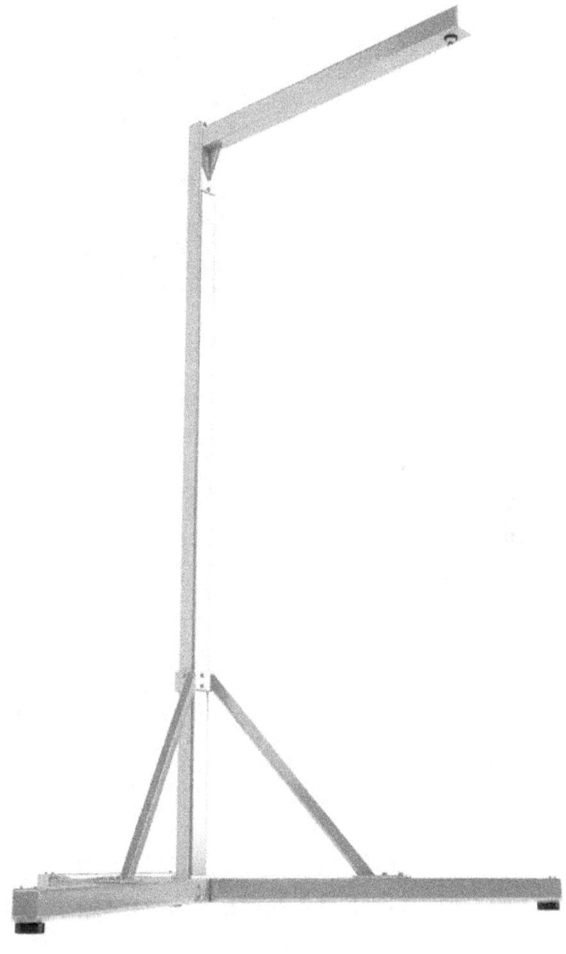

The only drawback to the bag stand is that it limits your ability to move 360 degrees around the double end bag.

Setting the Proper Height of the Bag

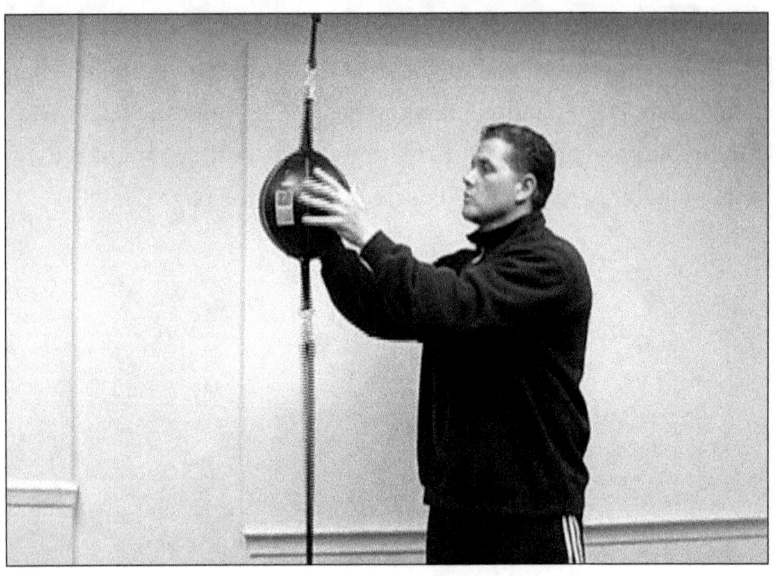

Once you hang the double end bag, the next important issue is making certain it is set at the proper height. One of the most common mistakes is setting the height of the bag too low.

Be sure that your bag is set up so that you can effectively land head level shots. This is especially important for people who intend on using the double end bag for self-defense or sports combat like mixed martial arts. Essentially, the top of the double end bag should be level with your head.

To ensure the proper height you might have to adjust the length of the elastic rubber cables or bungee straps. This will most likely take a bit of experimentation and some trial and error, but the result will be worth the effort.

The following photographs illustrate the best way to determine the proper hight of the double end bag.

Improper Bag Height

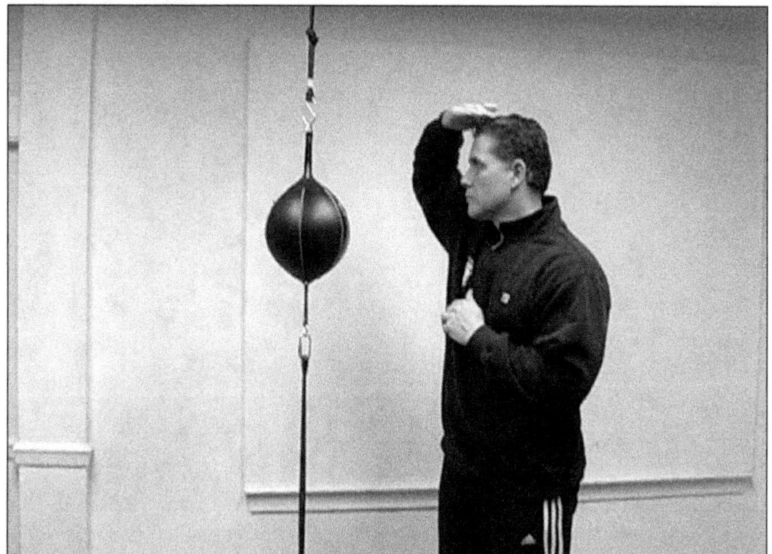

The following photographs demonstrate a double end bag that is set too low for effective training.

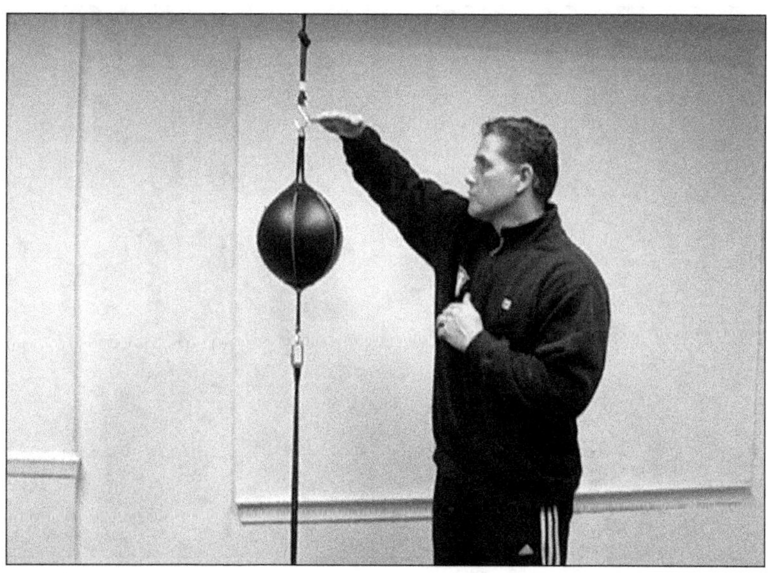

Notice how the top of the double end bag is not raised at head level.

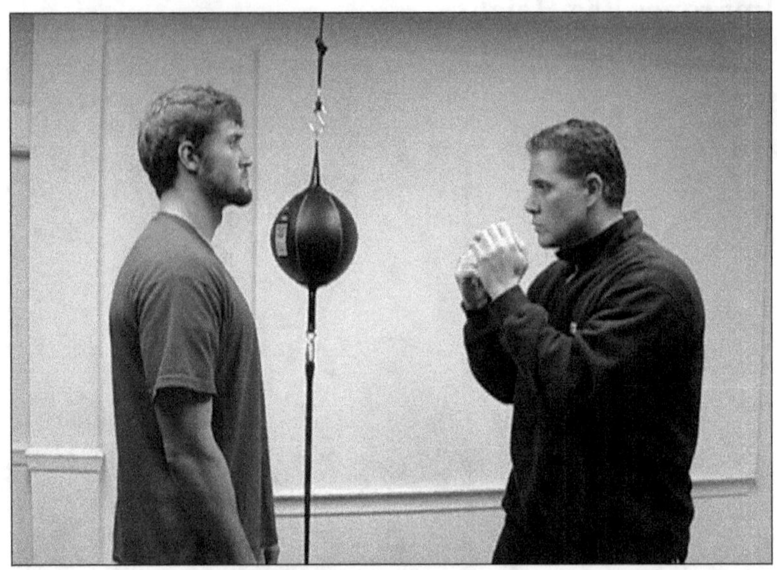

Once again, the following photographs demonstrate a double end bag that is set too low for effective training. Notice how the bag compares to the height of a real opponent.

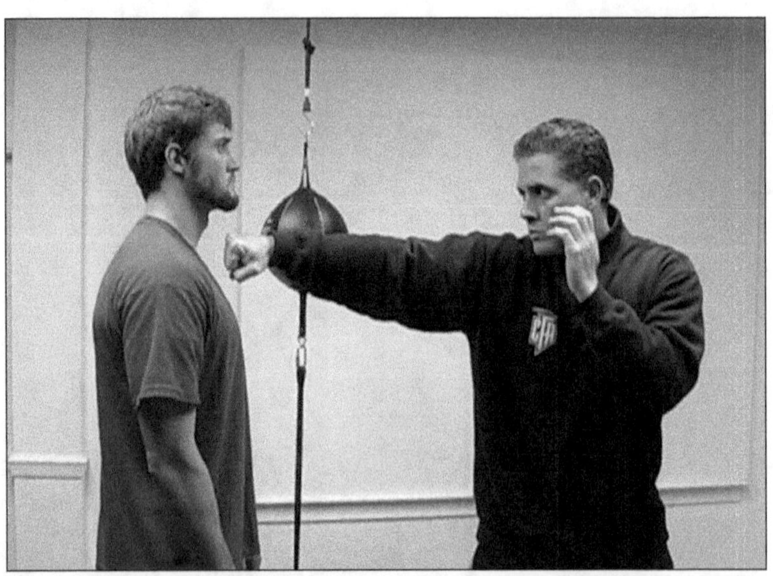

You won't be able to target realistic head shots if the double end bag is set too low. Instead, you'll be aiming for the opponent's throat and upper chest.

Proper Bag Height

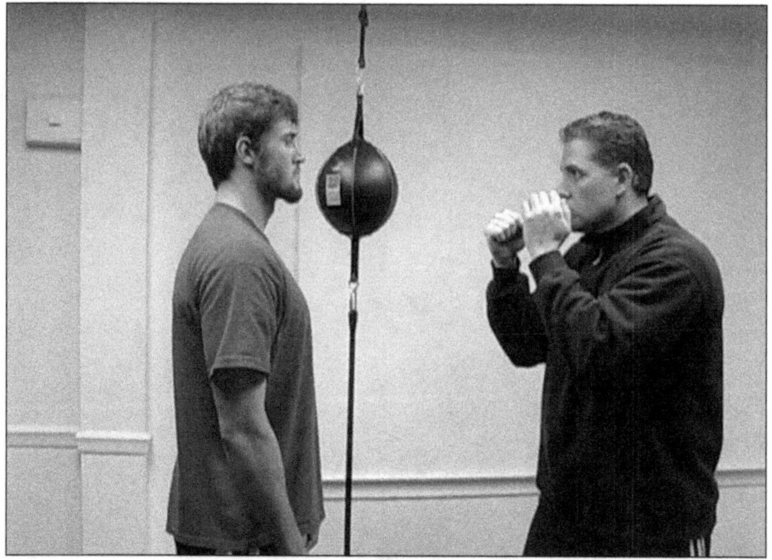

The following photographs demonstrate the correct height of a double end bag. Notice how the bag is raised to a realistic target height.

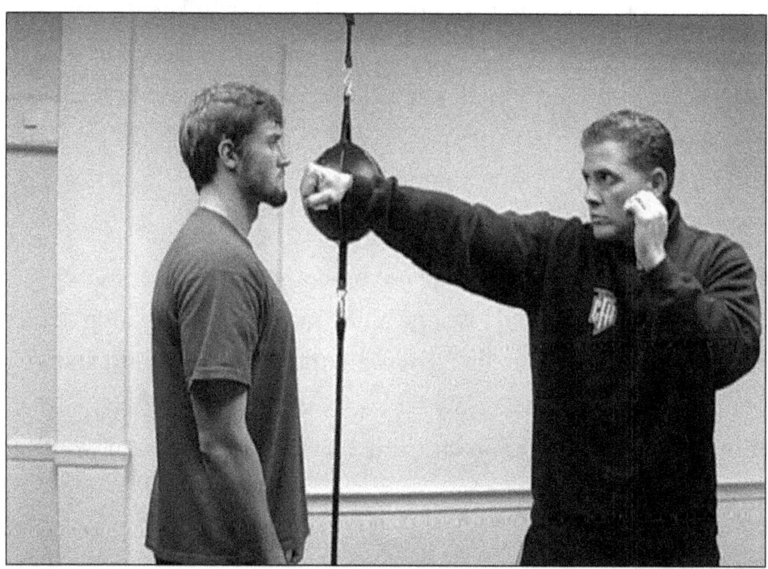

When set at the proper height, you will be able to target accurate head shots.

Air Pressure and Cable Tension

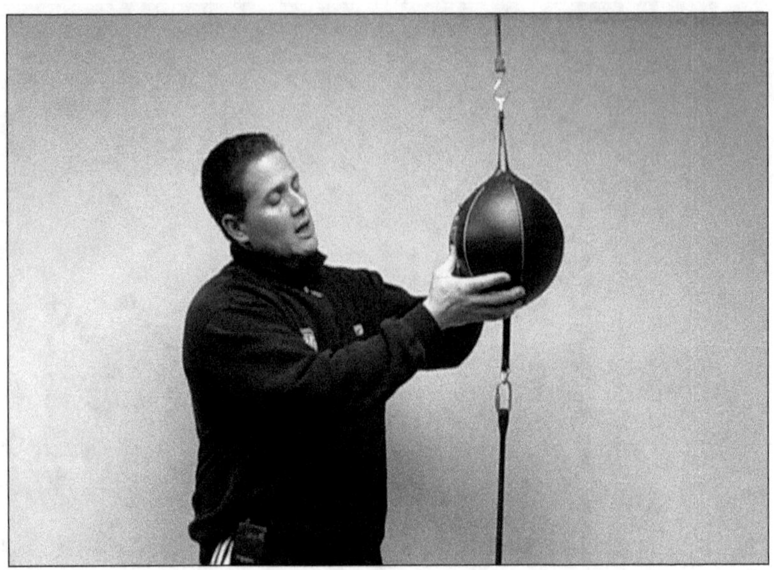

Air pressure is another important consideration when setting up the double end bag. It's important not to over-inflate the bag, for example, you don't want it to be rock-hard like a basketball. Essentially, you need a moderate amount of air pressure in the bag. You should be able to make a noticeable indentation in the bag when you press into it with your thumb .

The tension of the elastic rubber cables or bungee straps is also important. If the straps are too tight, the bag will not move unpredictably and you'll lose one of the major benefits of double end bag training. Remember, you want the bag to move fast and unpredictably. This means the cables should be relatively loose, allowing you to push it forward and stretch it out in front of you.

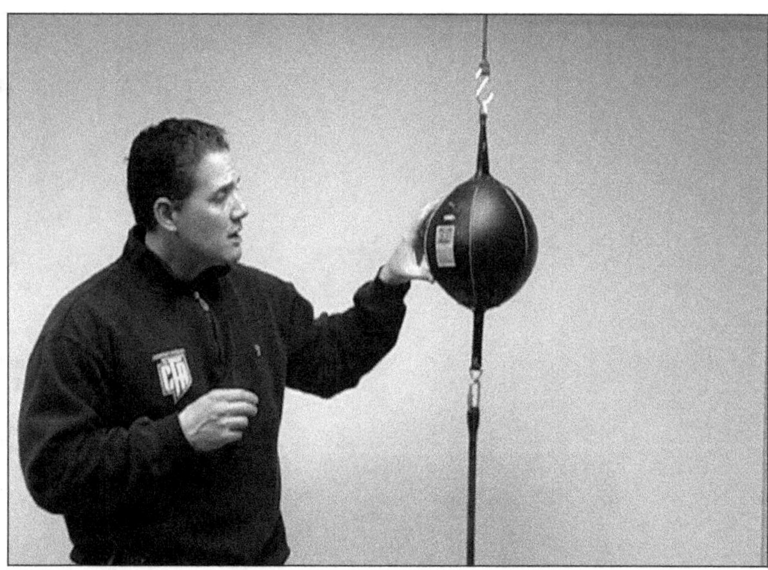

The best way to test the proper tension of the elastic rubber cables or bungee straps is to push it forward and stretch it out in front of you.

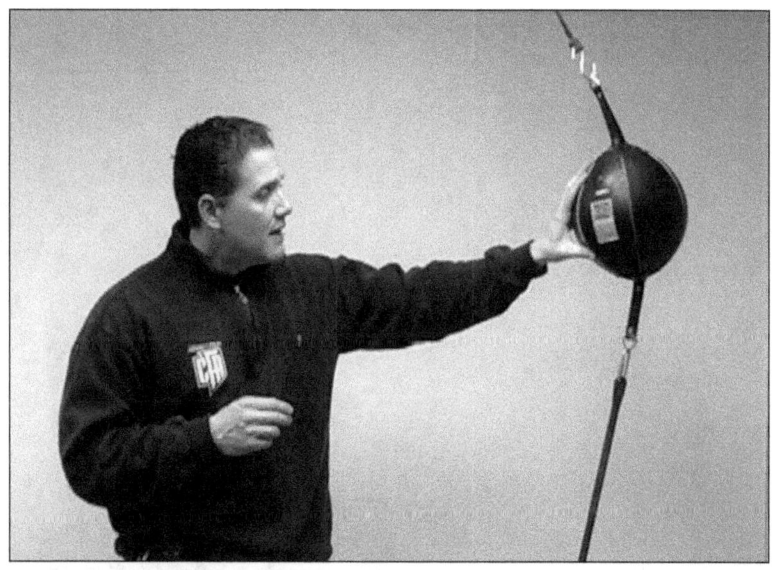

Here, Sammy Franco demonstrates the correct cable tension required for the double end bag.

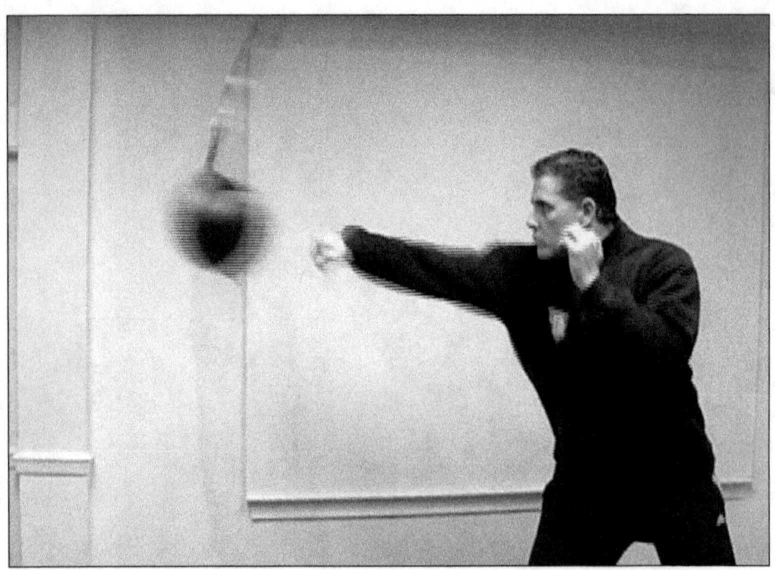

The correct amount of cable tension will permit the double end bag to quickly flex backwards when struck.

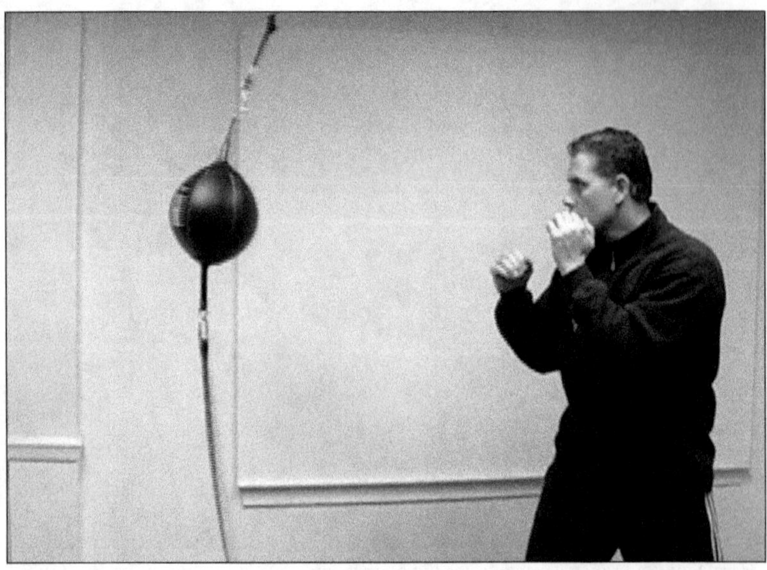

Setting the proper cable tension will also ensure the bag is responsive during training.

Double End Bag Safety Tips

Before you launch ahead and start hitting the bag, it's important to go over some important safety tips.

- Consult with your personal physician before beginning this or any other strenuous exercise program.
- Immediately stop training if you feel pain or discomfort.
- To avoid injuries, always begin your workout with a light round first.
- Never hold your breath when working out on the bag.
- Always remember to exhale when delivering a blow to the bag.
- Always keep your workout area clear of objects.
- While training, make certain that no one is standing near the bag. This includes pets.
- When setting up the double end bag, always follow the manufacturer's instructions.
- To avoid hyper-extending your arm, never strike the bag unless you sure you will make contact.
- Always warm up with light stretching before working out on the bag.
- Never hang your bag directly next to a window.
- Before you workout, always check and make certain the double end bag and its support structure is secure.
- Immediately replace worn parts such as elastic cables, hooks, snap links and other metal parts that wear out over time.
- When working out on the bag, always remember to keep both of your hands up at all times.

Double End Bag Workout

- Always wear loose fitting clothing when working out on the bag.
- To avoid injuring your hands and damaging your bag, never workout with rings or jewelry on your hands.
- Never strike the bag with full force until you have mastered the proper body mechanics.
- To avoid spraining or breaking your wrists, never bend your wrists when punching the bag.
- Don't strike the double end bag with bare knuckles, until your hands are conditioned to withstand the impact.
- Get into the habit of timing you workout rounds.
- Proper punching form is always more important than intensity.
- Never fully extend or "lock out" your arms when punching the bag.
- Depending on the type of punch that you are executing, always maintain the correct distance from the bag.
- Never allow people to pull or swing from the elastic cables.
- Avoid lifting your chin and exposing your centerline when working out on the bag.
- Maintain proper footwork and stay balanced at all times when working out on the double end bag.

Double End Bag Gear

If you want to get the most out of your workouts, you might want to invest in some gear. Here are just a few items you might want to consider purchasing to help you with your training.

Bag Gloves

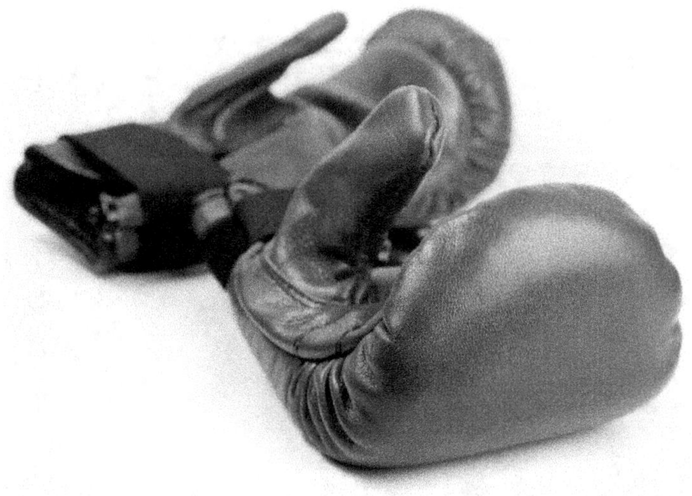

Bag gloves are lightweight gloves that offer excellent protection to your hands when working out on all types of punching bags. They are constructed of either top grain cowhide or durable vinyl. There are two styles of bag gloves sold on the market:

- *Mitt style gloves*
- *Finger style gloves*

Some of the mitt style bag gloves may also have a small metal bar sewn into the palm grip area to aid in fist stabilization. Bag glove sizes are usually small, medium, large and extra large.

When buying bag gloves, spare no expense and look for a reputable and high-quality brand. This will provide years of reliable use and will help ensure a better quality workout.

If you don't think you will need bag gloves, think again. Working out on the double end bag, without hand protection might causes sore knuckles, bruised bones, hand inflammation, sore wrists and bloody knuckles. Remember, if your hands are torn up from training, it will set your progress back for several weeks for your hands to completely heal.

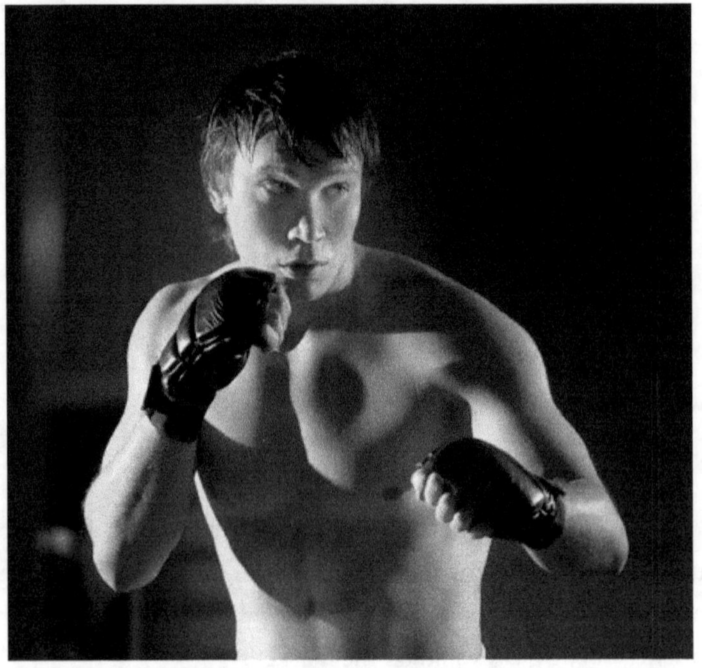

In this photo, finger style bag gloves.

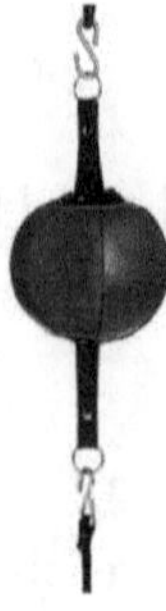

Bag gloves are strictly designed to protect your hands and fingers when working out. They don't stabilize your wrists when punching the bag.

Boxing Gloves

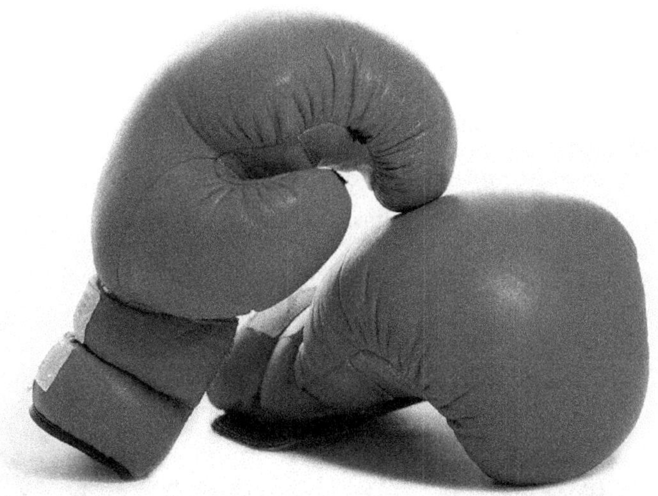

Compared to bag gloves, boxing gloves are heavier, significantly larger, and they are generally used for full-contact sparring and sports combat competition.

However, boxing gloves also can be used for double end bag training. In fact, boxing gloves are often used by advanced practitioners for developing strength and endurance in their shoulders and arms.

The ideal boxing glove is one that provides comfort, protection, and durability. Depending on your training objective, the glove can weigh anywhere from ten to sixteen ounces.

Here are some important features to be aware of when purchasing a pair of boxing gloves:

- To avoid wrist injuries, you want the glove to fit snugly around your hand.
- The glove should be composed of multi-layered foam padding.

- The glove should have a sufficient palm grip that provides comfort and fist stabilization.
- To avoid a thumb injury, the glove should have thumb-lock stitching.
- The glove should be double-stitched to ensure durability.
- The entire glove should be constructed of top quality materials to increase its durability.
- The glove should be relatively easy to slip-on and off your hands. Velcro fasteners are sometimes preferred over laces.

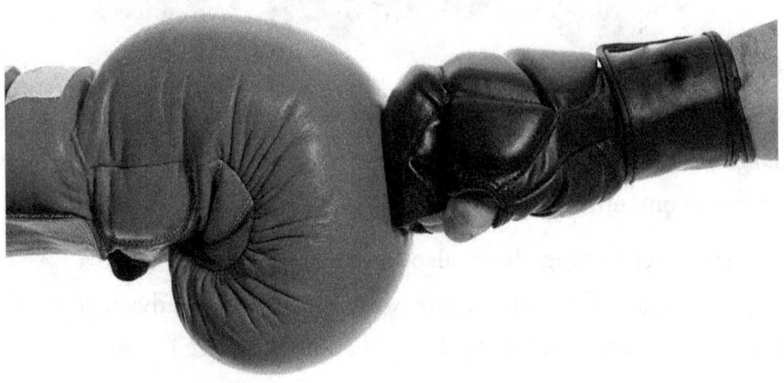

As you can see, there's a big difference between the bag glove (right) and the boxing glove (left).

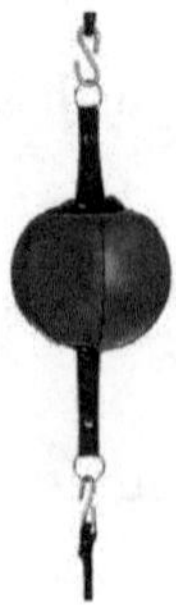

Boxing gloves can also be used if your knuckles are too sore or bruised to hit the bag with regular bag gloves. The extra padding can make all the difference between skipping a workout and sticking with your routine.

Hand Wraps

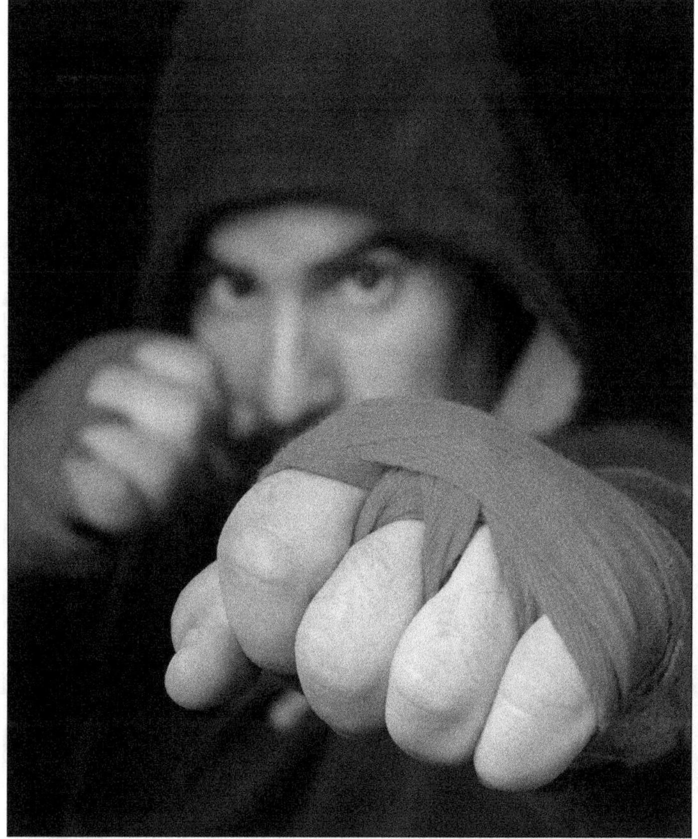

Hand Wraps (also called wrist wraps) are used by experienced athletes who want an added measure of protection to their hands and wrists when hitting the double end bag. They provide support to the entire hand and wrist area and can help prevent osteoarthritis in later years.

Essentially, hand wraps are long strips of cloth measuring two inches wide and nine to eighteen feet long. The longer hand wraps are more often used by practitioners who have large hands and who wish to have greater hand protection. You can find hand wraps at most sporting goods stores as well as the Internet.

Hand wraps should be used in conjunction with either large bag gloves or boxing gloves, however some practitioners prefer to strike the double end bag with just the hand wraps.

Hand wraps are washable and should be cleaned after every workout. Although there are many hand wrapping techniques, the procedures shown on the next page is suggested.

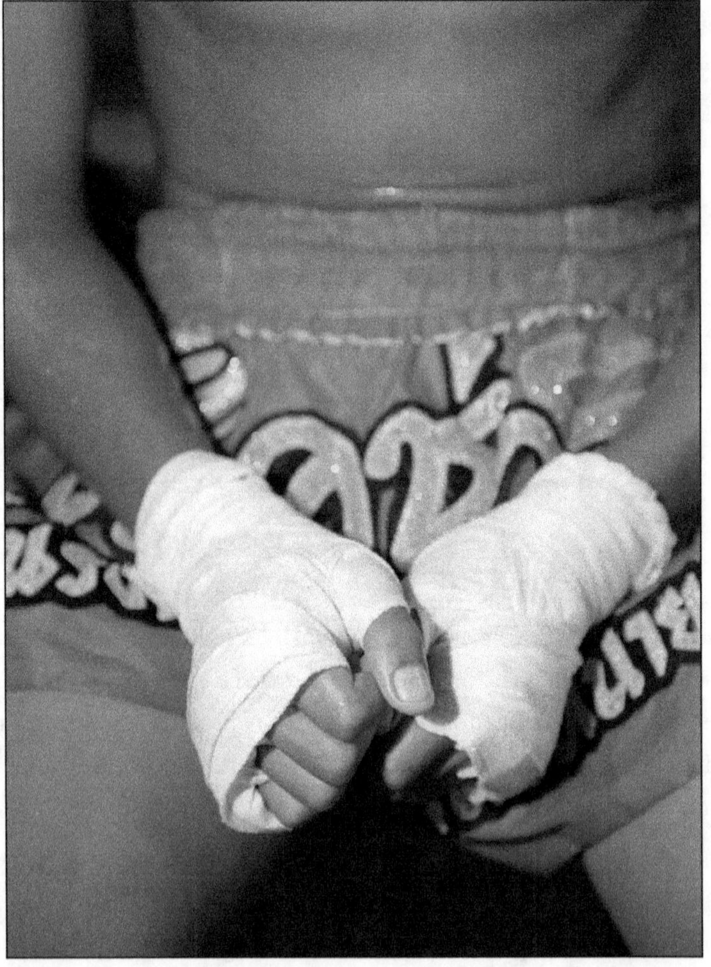

Hand wraps are used all over the world and by many cultures. Here, a Muay Thai fighter takes a break during his training.

How to Apply Hand and Wrist Wraps

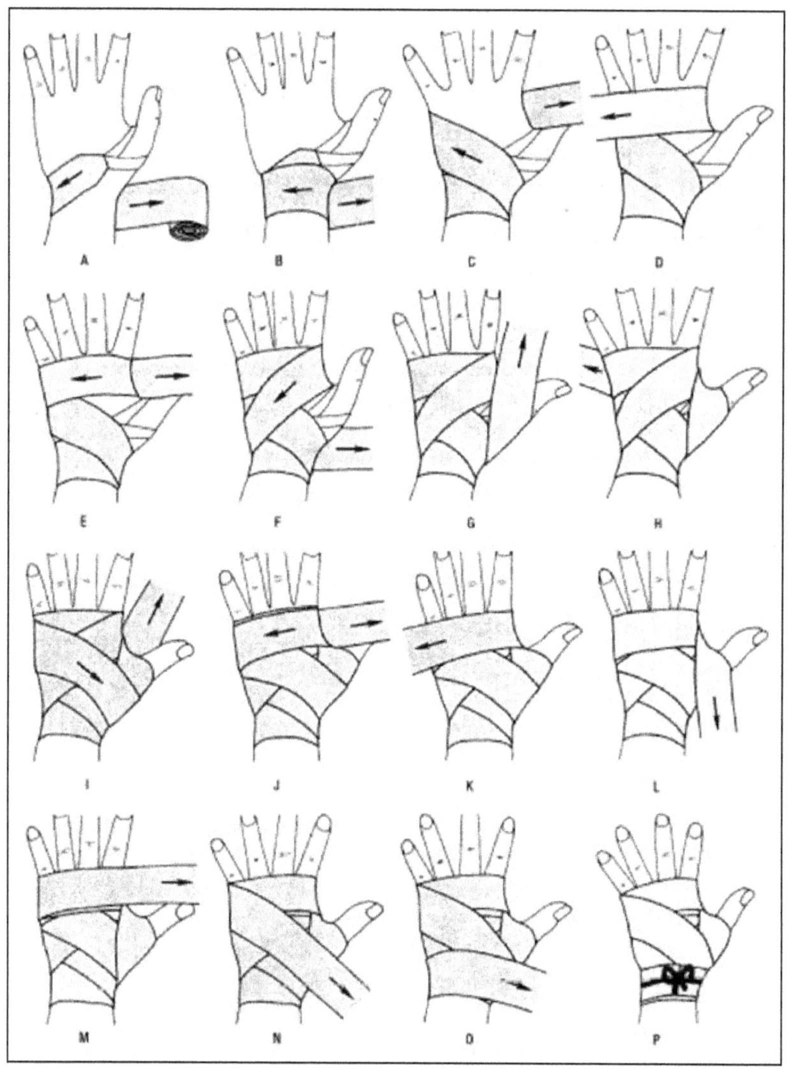

How to wrap your hands and wrists with hand wraps. Follow steps A through P

Interval Workout Timer

Since double end bag training is structured around time and rounds, you should invest in a good workout timer. Boxers, mixed martial artists, and kickboxers will use workout timers to keep track of their time during their rounds.

Most workout timers will allow you to adjust your round lengths anywhere from 30 seconds to 9 minutes. Rest time can be set from 30 seconds to 5 minutes depending on your level of conditioning and training goals.

There are several professional timers sold on the market, and they vary in price. Be forewarned! Some of them can be very pricey. However, there are numerous smartphone apps that replicate the same function and characteristics of an actual interval timer. These workout timer apps are convenient and very inexpensive. Your best bet is to search the Internet or your favorite app store for one that meets your specific needs.

Workout Timers are great for:

- Keeping track of the number of rounds and the time of each round.
- Measuring your current level of cardiovascular conditioning.
- Monitoring your progress in your training.
- Creating healthy competition in your workout routine.

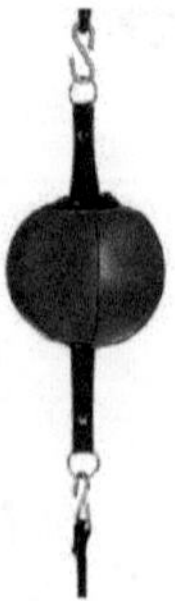

One final reminder before moving on to the next chapter, double end bag training can be very demanding on the heart. Before you begin any workout program, including those suggested in this book, it is important to check with your physician to see if you have any condition that might be aggravated by strenuous exercise.

Chapter 3
The Fighting Stance and Footwork

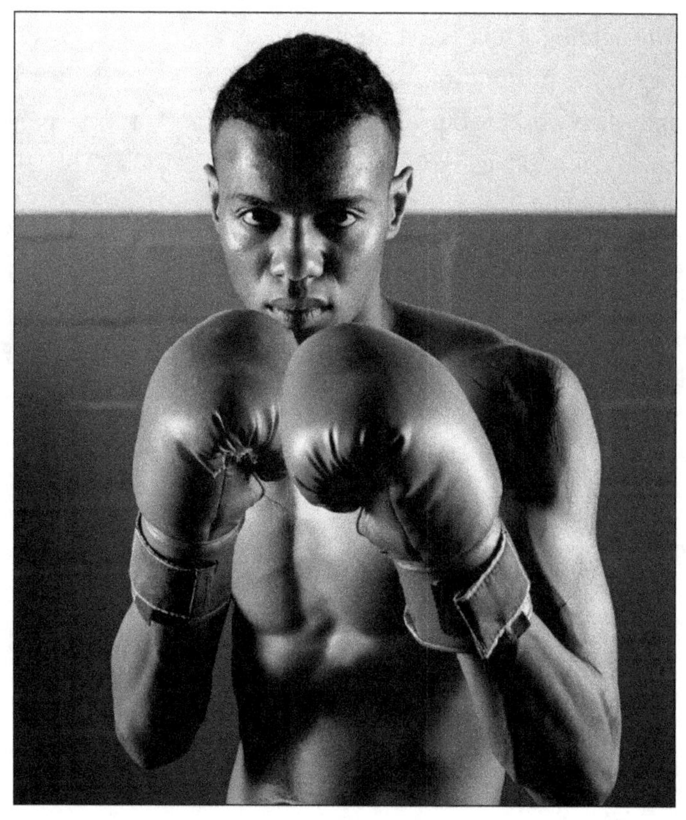

The Fighting Stance

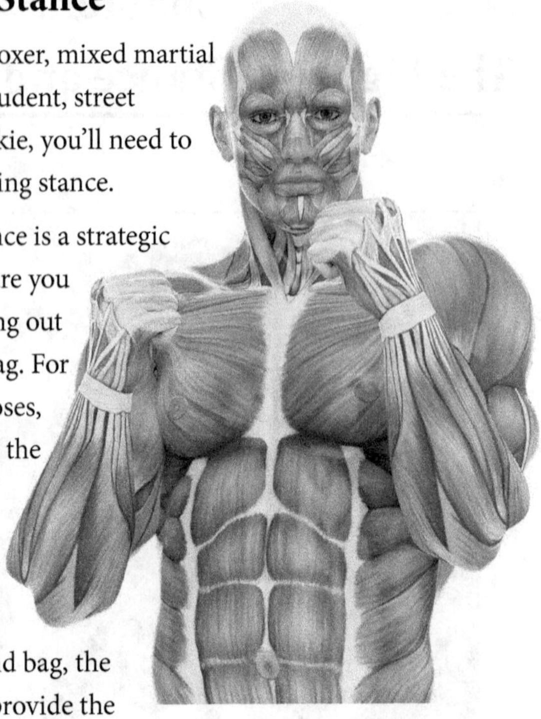

Whether you are a boxer, mixed martial artist, self-defense student, street fighter or fitness junkie, you'll need to learn about the fighting stance.

The fighting stance is a strategic and aggressive posture you assume when working out on the double end bag. For all intents and purposes, the fighting stance is the foundation for all of your punching and striking techniques.

When working out on the double end bag, the fighting stance will provide the following:

- **Speed**
- **Striking power**
- **Stability**
- **Mobility**
- **Balance**
- **Offensive fluidity**
- **Maximizes limb extension**
- **Complete visual picture**

The fighting stance is not only used for bag training. In fact, the fighting stance is used for both offensive and defensive purposes during actual combat. It stresses strategic soundness and simplicity over complexity and style. The fighting stance also facilitates maximum execution of punches, kicks and strikes while simultaneously protecting your targets against possible counter attacks from the opponent.

The Centerline

One of the most important considerations of a fighting stance is the centerline. Your centerline is an imaginary vertical line that divides your body in half. Located on this line are some of your most vital impact targets. This includes your eyes, nose, chin, throat, solar plexus, and groin.

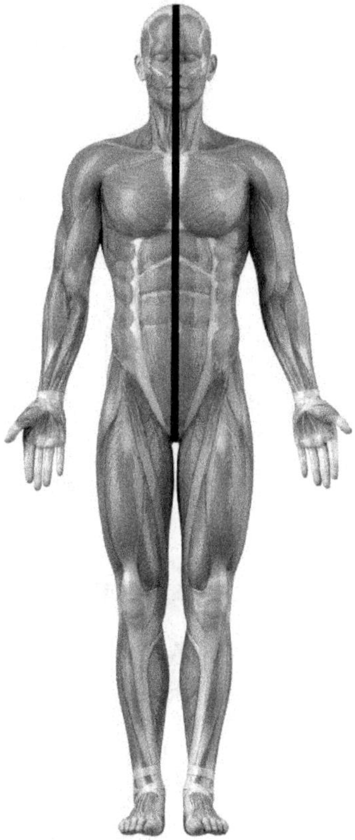

The Centerline

Centerline Placement

The proper placement of your centerline (in relation to the double end bag) is critical and will directly effect the following:

1. Target Exposure - A properly positioned centerline will minimize the number of anatomical targets exposed to the bag when working out.

2. Balance - A properly positioned centerline will maximize your balance and stability during your workout. This is especially important when delivering explosive combination attacks.

3. Mobility - A properly positioned centerline will also maximize your ability to move quickly and efficiently around the bag.

4. Power Generation - A properly angled centerline permits maximum hip and shoulder rotation which translates to greater impact power when throwing punches, strikes, and other blows at the bag. For example, try throwing a punch at the bag with both of your feet planted squarely in front of you? Notice anything? There's no snap to the punch, of course.

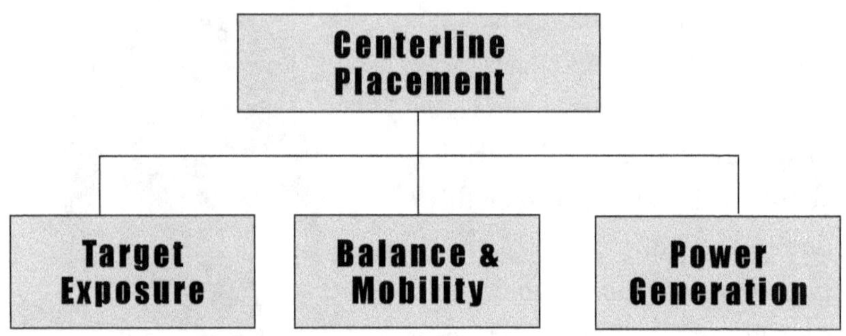

Your centerline placement will have a direct effect on the following factors.

How To Assume a Fighting Stance

Essentially, there are two variations of the fighting stance, the orthodox and southpaw. Let's begin with the orthodox stance.

To assume the orthodox stance, place the left side of your body forward and closest to the double end bag. Then, blade your feet and centerline at approximately forty-five degrees from your bag. Make certain to place your feet approximately a shoulder-width apart with both of your knees bent and flexible.

Mobility is also important, as we'll discuss later. All footwork and strategic movement should be performed on the balls of your feet. Your weight distribution is also an important factor. Since double end bag training is dynamic, your weight distribution will frequently change. However, when stationary, keep 50 percent of your body weight on each leg and always be in control of it.

Next, the hands are aligned one behind the other along your centerline. The lead arm is held high and bent at approximately 90 degrees. The rear arm is kept back by the chin. Arranged this way, the hands not only protect the upper centerline but also allow quick deployment of your punches as well as other striking techniques.

When holding your guard, do not tighten your shoulder or arm muscles prior to striking. Stay relaxed and loose. Finally, keep your chin slightly angled down. This diminishes target size and reduces the likelihood of a paralyzing blow to your chin or a lethal strike to your throat during an actual self-defense encounter.

If you want to assume a southpaw fighting stance, you would perform the very same steps mentioned above but with your right side facing forward and closest to the bag. Generally, most right handed people with use the orthodox stance, while left handed people will opt for the southpaw.

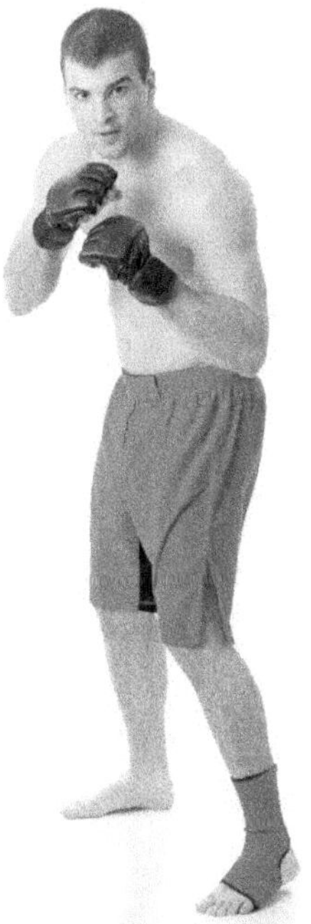

The Orthodox Fighting Stance.

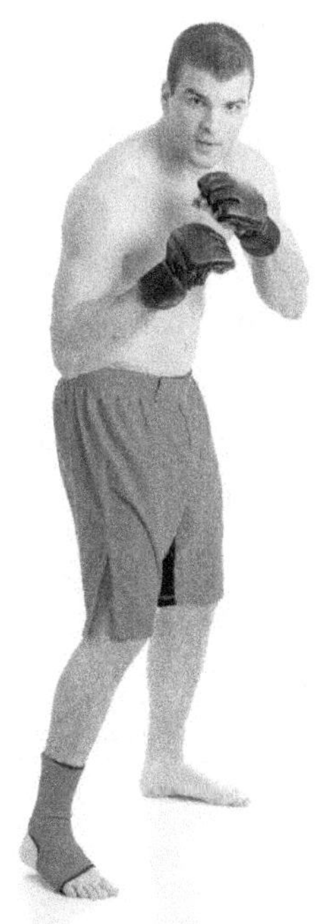

The Southpaw Fighting Stance.

Double End Bag Workout

However, for those who are interested in reality based self-defense, you must be able to fight your adversary with equal ability on both the right and left sides of your body. This means that you would need to practice double end bag work from both the southpaw and orthodox stances.

The best method for practicing your fighting stance is in front of a full-length mirror. Place the mirror in an area that allows sufficient room for movement; a garage or basement is perfect. Stand in front of the mirror, far enough away to see your entire body. Stand naturally with your arms relaxed at your sides. Now close your eyes and quickly assume your fighting stance. Open your eyes and check for flaws. Look for low hand guards, improper foot positioning or body angle, rigid shoulders and knees, etc. Drill this way repeatedly, working from both the right and left side. Practice this until your fighting stance becomes second nature.

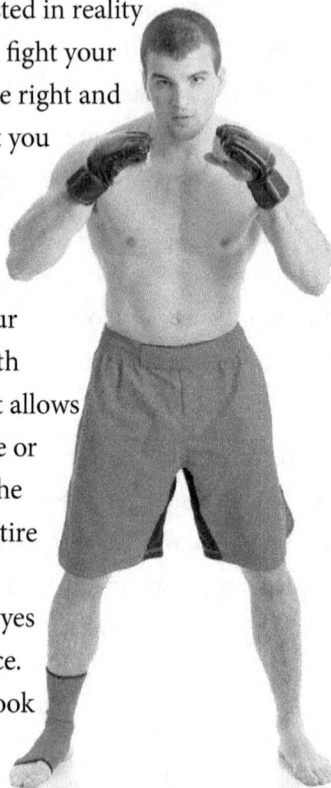

One common mistake beginners make is to stand squarely in front of the double end bag without regard to their stance. Never stand squarely in front of the bag. Not only will this expose your centerline targets, it also diminishes your balance, inhibits efficient footwork, and minimizes your reach.

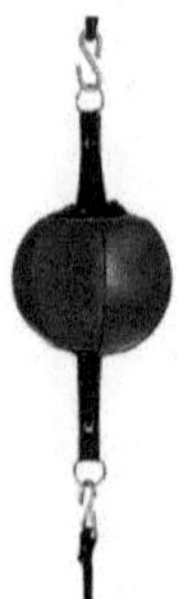

A full-length mirror can also be used for shadow boxing training. Shadow boxing is the creative deployment of offensive and defensive techniques and maneuvers against an imaginary opponent.

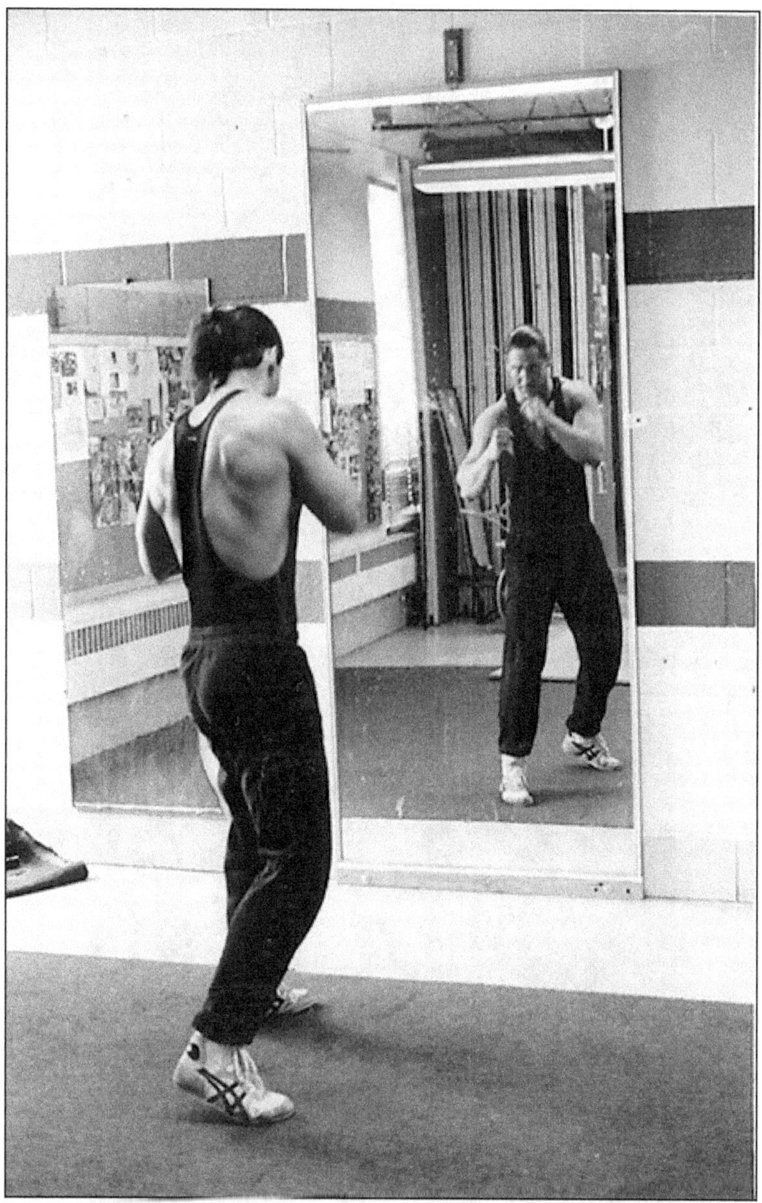

Pictured here, one of Mr. Franco's students warming up in front of the mirror before his double end bag workout.

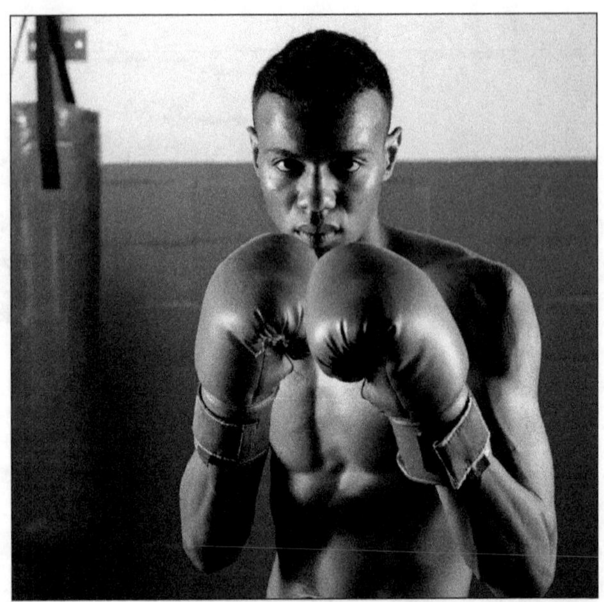

Pictured here, the classic "boxer's stance." Notice how the fighter's centerline is angled at approximately 45-degrees.

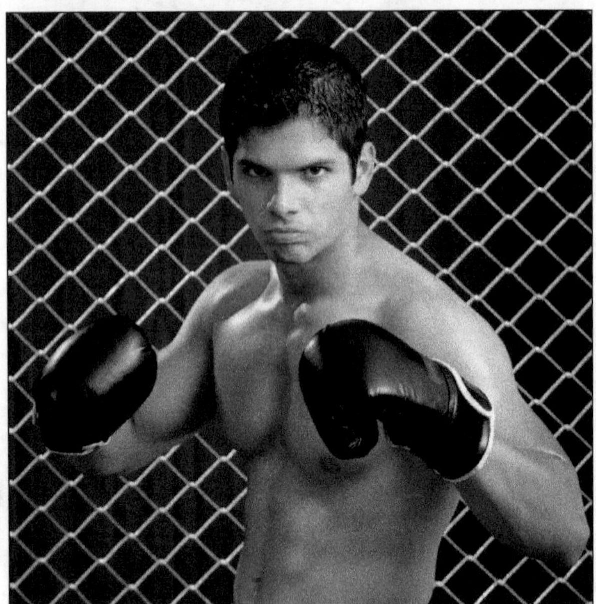

Avoid the tendency to let both your elbows flair out to the sides. This type of elbow positioning places your hands away from proper body mechanic alignment.

Fighting Stance Review

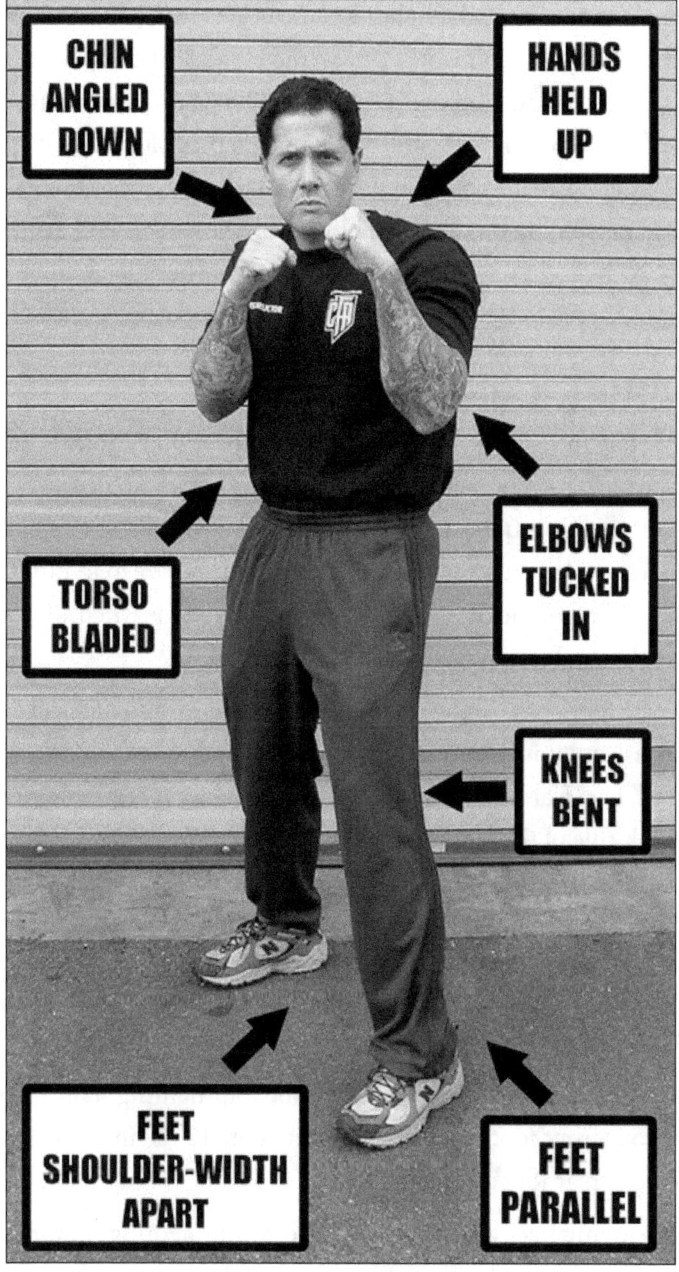

You'll Need to Move Around the Bag!

Now that we have the fighting stance covered, it's time to talk about mobility and footwork. One of the biggest mistakes beginners make when working out on the double end bag, is to just stand in front of it and beat it to death! While this methodology might have some limited street fighting applications, it should not be your sole method of training on the bag. Remember, the double end bag must swing freely, and this means that you must also be able to move with it.

Footwork & Mobility

I define mobility as the ability to move your body quickly and freely, which is accomplished through basic footwork. The safest footwork involves quick, economical steps performed on the balls of your feet, while you remain relaxed and balanced. Keep in mind that balance is one of the most important considerations when working out on the double end bag.

Basic footwork can be used for both offensive and defensive purposes, and it is structured around four general directions: forward, backward, right, and left. However, always remember this footwork rule of thumb: ***Always move the foot closest to the direction you want to go first, and let the other foot follow an equal distance.*** This prevents cross-stepping, which can be disastrous in a high-risk combat situation.

Basic Footwork Movements

1. Moving forward (advance)- from your fighting stance, first move your front foot forward (approximately 12 -18 inches) and then move your rear foot an equal distance.

2. Moving backward (retreat) - from your fighting stance, first move your rear foot backward (approximately 12 - 18 inches) and then move your front foot an equal distance.

3. Moving right (sidestep right) - from your fighting stance, first move your right foot to the right (approximately 12 - 18 inches) and then move your left foot an equal distance.

4. Moving left (sidestep left) - from your fighting stance, first move your left foot to the left (approximately 12 - 18 inches) and then move your right foot an equal distance.

Practice these four movements for 10 to 15 minutes a day in front of a full-length mirror. In a couple weeks, your footwork should be quick, balanced, and natural.

Circling Right and Left

Strategic circling is an advanced form of footwork where you will use your front leg as a pivot point. This type of movement permits you to move 360-degrees around the bag and also allow you to strike from various angles. Strategic circling can be performed from either a left or right stance.

Circling left (from a left stance) - this means you'll be moving your body around the double end bag in a clockwise direction. From a left stance, step 8 to 12 inches to the left with your left foot, then use your left leg as a pivot point and wheel your entire rear leg to the left until the correct stance and positioning is acquired.

Circling right (from a right stance) - from a right stance, step 8 to 12 inches to the right with your right foot, then use your right leg as a pivot point and wheel your entire rear leg to the right until the correct stance and positioning is acquired.

Avoid Cross-Stepping When Hitting The Bag

Cross-stepping is the process of crossing one foot in front or behind the other when moving around the bag. Such sloppy footwork makes you vulnerable to a variety of problems. Some include:

- It severely compromises your balance.
- It restricts the offensive flow of punching.
- It limits quick and rapid footwork.
- It can lead to a sprained ankle.

As I said earlier, the best way to avoid cross-stepping is to follow this basic footwork rule of thumb: ***Always move the foot closest to the direction you want to go first, and let the other foot follow an equal distance.***

Explosive Footwork

Explosive footwork is another important component of double end bag training. In fact, this type of dynamic movement plays a vital role in both offensive and defensive fighting. In offense, explosive footwork allows you to rush your target and maintain a devastating

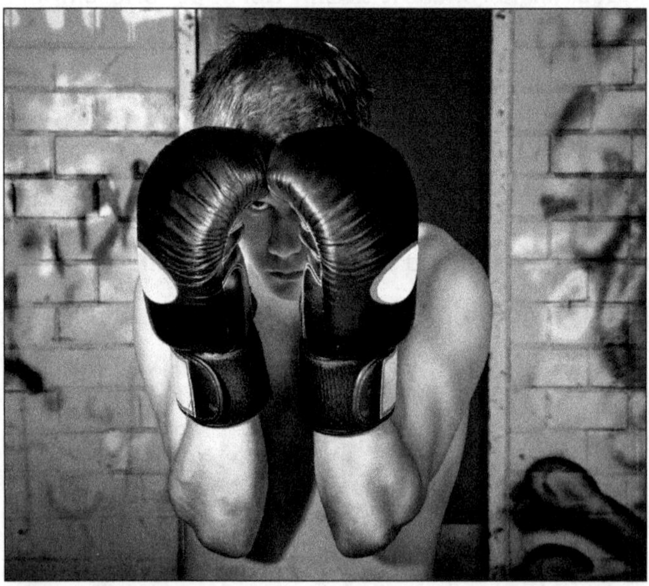

Try to visualize the double end bag as a living breathing opponent who will hit back the moment you let your guard down.

compound attack. In defense, it permits you to disengage quickly from the range of an overwhelming assault.

Explosive footwork is predicated on the following five important factors. They include the following:

1. **Basic footwork** - you must first master the basic footwork skills before incorporating ballistic movements.
2. **Proper body posture** - maintaining correct body posture through footwork movements will prevent loss of balance.
3. **Powerful legs**- strong and powerful upper and lower legs will allow you to launch your body effortlessly through the ranges of combat.
4. **Equal weight distribution** - a noncommittal weight distribution (fifty percent on each leg) will permit you to move instantly in any direction.
5. **Raised heel** - this creates a springlike effect in your footwork movements.

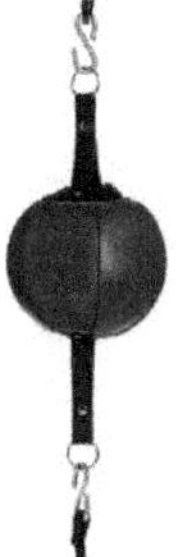

Although there are many components of efficient footwork, moving on the balls of your feet is vital. Flat-footed footwork will slow you down considerably during your bag training.

Double End Bag Workout

Chapter 4
The Art of Punching

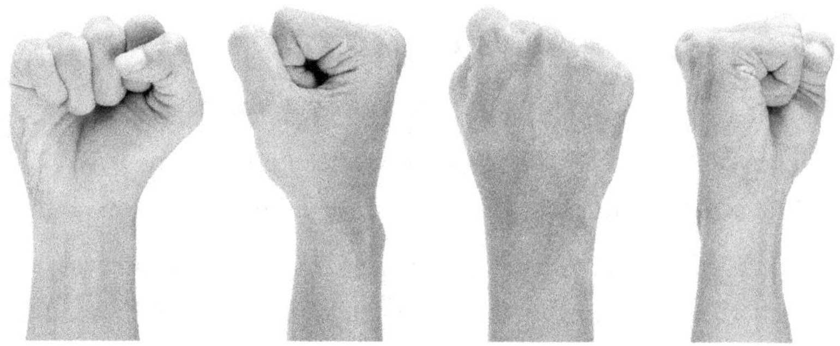

Injury Free Punching

Since the majority of your double end bag techniques will be delivered with your fists, it's essential that you know how to punch without sustaining a hand injury. Essentially, this requires you to understand and ultimately master a few concepts and body mechanic principles. Keep in mind that you do not have to be a professional boxer or martial arts expert to master these fundamental principles.

What Causes Hand Injuries?

There are four main causes of punching related hand injuries. They are incorrect fist configuration, skeletal misalignment, weak hands, wrist and forearms and hitting the wrong anatomical target.

While there are different body mechanics for each and every punch, there are four things that must take place to avoid a hand injury, when hitting the bag. They include the following:

- **Knowing how to make a proper fist.**
- **Possessing strong hands, wrists, and forearms.**
- **Maintaining skeletal alignment when striking the bag.**
- **Pinpoint target accuracy.**

How to Make a Proper Fist

The first thing you need to do is learn the proper way make a fist. It's ironic that some of the most experienced fighters don't know how to make a proper fist. As you can imagine, improper fist clenching can be disastrous for some of the following reasons:

- **You can jam, sprain, or break your fingers.**
- **You can destroy wrist alignment, resulting in a sprained or broken wrist.**

- **You'll lose significant impact power when hitting the bag.**

To make a proper fist, make sure your fingers are tightly clenched and that your thumb is securely wrapped around your second and third knuckles. Your fist should resemble a solid brick. Remember, if you cannot make a proper fist, you will not be capable of delivering a solid punch on the double end bag!

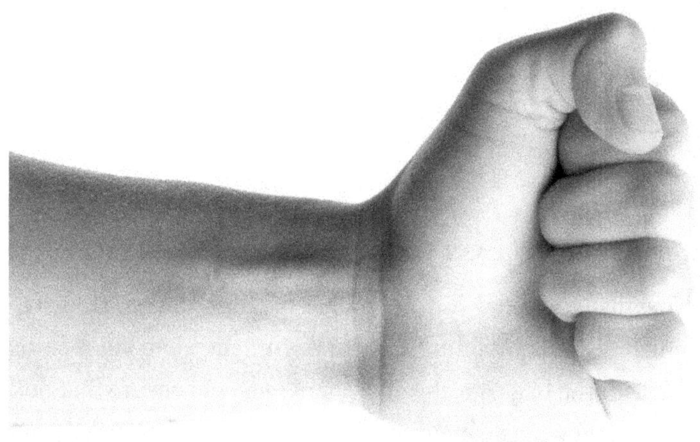

Pictured here, the correct way to make a fist.

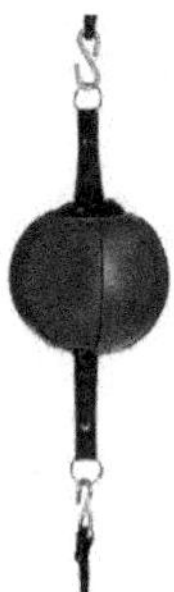

Long fingernails will compromise the structural integrity of your punch by causing your individual fingers to protrude from your fist. This can easily lead to a severe hand or wrist injury. If you are serious about training, consider keeping all of your fingernails very short.

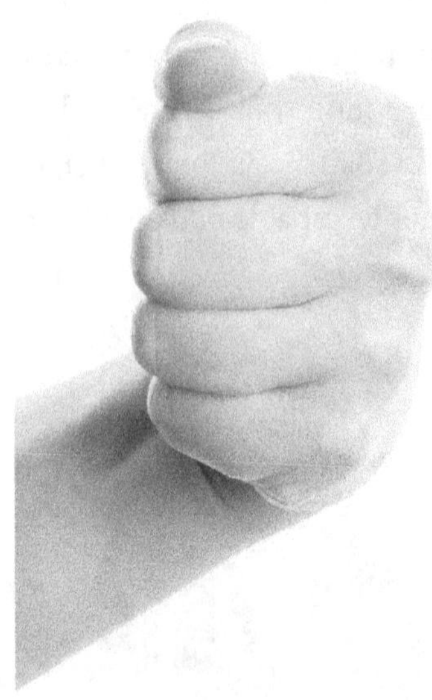

One of the biggest mistakes beginners make when making a fist is allowing their thumbs to protrude outward. This hand position is dangerous and can often lead to hand and finger injuries as well as powerless blows. Remember, always to keep your thumbs tightly wrapped around the other two fingers when throwing punches.

You Must Keep Everything Straight

Now that you know how to make a proper fist, your next step is learning how to maintaining skeletal alignment when your fist makes contact with the bag. Skeletal alignment will help ensure that both your hand and wrists will not buckle and break during impact with the double end bag.

Center Knuckle Contact

In order to maintain skeletal alignment when punching, you need to learn to punch with your center knuckle first. Punching with the center of your knuckle is important because it affords proper alignment and maximizes the impact of your blow.

Excluding hammer fist strikes, every conceivable punch (i.e., jab, rear cross, hook, uppercut, shovel hook, etc) can be delivered with center knuckle contact.

Center knuckle contact also prevents a broken hand or *boxer's fracture* from occurring. Essentially, a boxer's fracture occurs when the small metacarpal bone bends downward and toward the palm of the hand during impact with an extremely hard surface (such as a brick wall or human skull).

Contrary to what most karate schools teach, I suggest that you avoid striking the double end bag with your first two knuckles. This karate style of punching diffuses the weight transfer of the punch which can easily lead to a broken hand.

Wrist and Forearm Alignment

If you want to avoid breaking or spraining your wrists, you must always remember to keep your wrists aligned with your forearm throughout the execution of your punch. This applies to both linear punches (jab, rear cross) as well as circular punches (hooks, uppercuts, and shovel hooks.)

If your wrist bends or collapses on impact, you will either sprain or break it. It's that simple. Remember, a sprained or broken wrist will set back your bag training for weeks or months.

Also, don't make the false assumption that boxing gloves or hands wraps will always keep your wrists straight. I know of several cases where people actually sprained their wrists while wearing both hand wraps and boxing gloves.

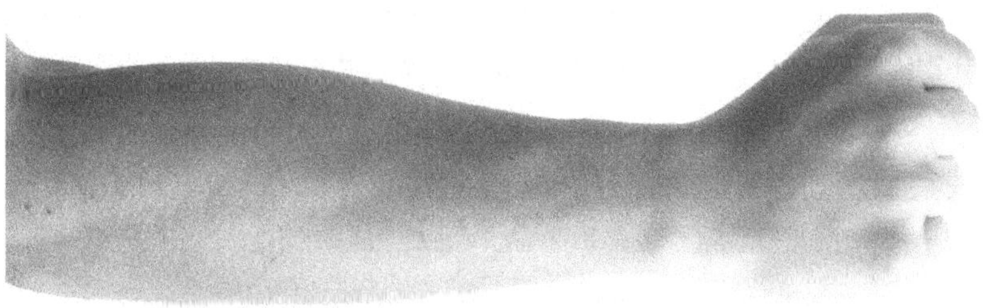

If you want to avoid breaking or spraining your wrists, you must always remember to keep your wrists aligned with your forearm throughout the execution of your punch.

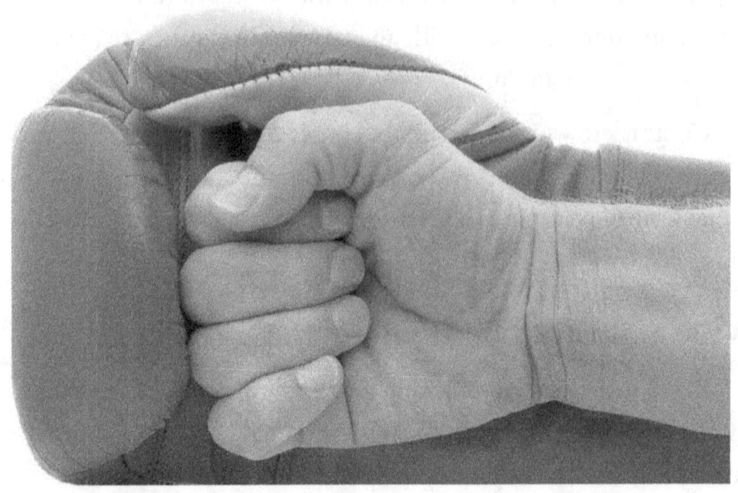

Don't make the false assumption that boxing gloves or bag gloves will keep your wrists straight. I can assure you, they won't.

One of the best ways to learn how to throw a punch without bending your wrists is to regularly workout on the heavy bag. The heavy bag will provide the necessary amount of resistance to progressively strengthen and condition the bones, tendons and ligaments in your wrists. Just remember to start off slowly and gradually increase the force of your punches.

Strong Hands, Wrists and Forearms

Proper fist configuration and wrist alignment are critical, but that is really only half of the equation. You must have strong hands, wrists, and forearms to withstand the actual force of impact.

You will, therefore, need to perform specific hand and forearm exercises to strengthen these muscles. Bruce Lee was well aware of this important fact. As a matter of fact, he would religiously strengthen and develop his hands and forearms for the rigors of power punching. Lee knew that powerful and injury free punching depends largely on the overall strength and structural integrity of your hands, wrists and forearms.

Conditioning and Strength Training

There are many efficient ways of strengthening your hands, wrists and forearms for double end bag training. If you are low on cash and just starting out, you can begin by squeezing a tennis ball a couple times per week. One hundred repetitions per hand would be a good start.

Power Putty

Later on you can add power putty to your hand strengthening routine. This unique hand exerciser is made up of silicone rubber that can be squeezed, pulled, pinched, clawed and stretched in just about any conceivable direction. This tough, resistant putty will strengthen the muscles of your forearm, wrists, hands and fingers.

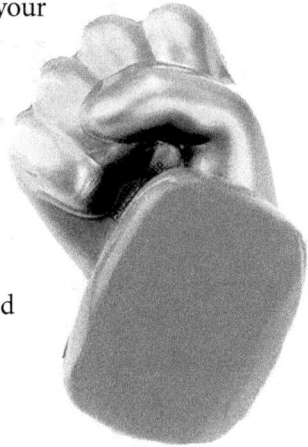

Hand Grippers

Another quick and effective way to strengthen your hands, wrists and forearms is to work out with heavy duty hand grippers. While there are a wide selection of them on the market, I prefer using the Captains of Crush brand. These high-quality grippers are virtually indestructible and they come in a variety of different resistance levels ranging from 60 to 365 pounds.

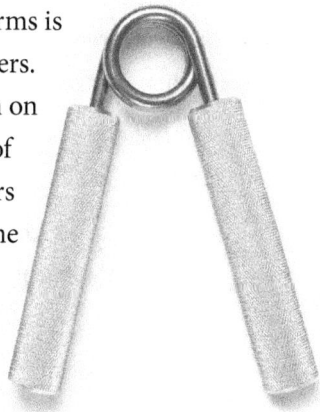

Weight Training

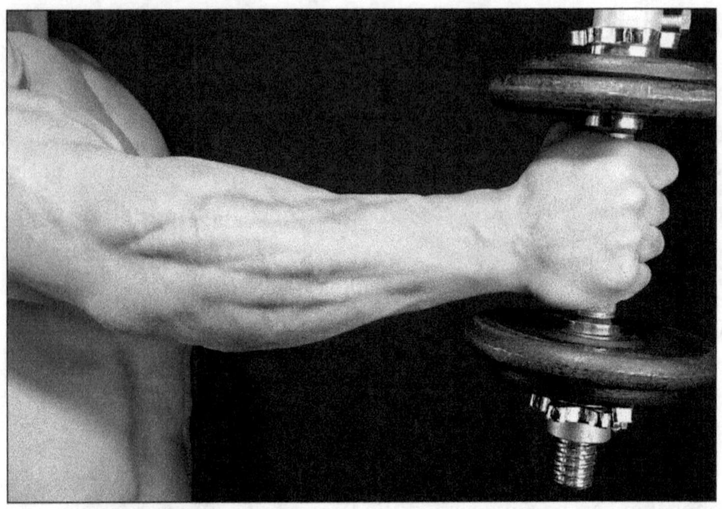

Finally, you can condition your wrists and forearms by performing various forearm exercises with free weights. Exercises like hammer curls, reverse curls, wrist curls, and reverse wrist curls are great for developing strong wrists, forearms, and hands. When training your forearms, be sure to work both your extensor and flexor muscles. Here are a few to get you started:

Barbell Wrist Curls

This exercise strengthens the flexor muscles. Perform 5 sets of 8-10 repetitions. To perform the exercise, follow these steps:

1. Sit at the end of a bench, grab a barbell with an underhand grip and place both of your hands close together.
2. In a smooth and controlled fashion, slowly bend your wrists and lower the barbell toward the floor.
3. Contract your forearms and curl the weight back to the starting position.

Reverse Wrist Curls

This exercise develops and strengthens the extensor muscle of the forearm. Perform 6 sets of 6-8 repetitions. To perform the exercise, follow these steps:

1. Sit at the end of a bench, hold a barbell with an overhand grip (your hands should be approximately 11 inches apart) and place your forearms on top of your thighs.
2. Slowly lower the barbell as far as your wrists will allow.
3. Flex your wrists upward back to the starting position.

Behind-the-Back Wrist Curls

This exercise strengthens both the flexor muscles of the forearms. Perform 5 sets of 6-8 repetitions To perform the exercise, follow these steps:

1. Hold a barbell behind your back at arm's length (your hands should be approximately shoulder-width apart).
2. Uncurl your finger and let the barbell slowly roll down your palms.
3. Close your hands and roll the barbell back into your hands.

Hammer Curls

This exercise strengthens both the Brachialis and Brachioradialis muscles. Perform 5 sets of 8-10 repetitions. To perform the exercise, follow these steps:

1. Stand with both feet approximately shoulder-width apart, with both dumbbells at your sides.
2. Keeping your elbows close to your body and your palms facing inward, slowly curl both dumbbells upward towards your shoulders.

3. Slowly return to the starting position.

Reverse Barbell Curls

Reverse curls can be a great alternative to hammer curls. This exercise strengthens both the Brachialis and Brachioradialis muscles. Perform 5 sets of 8-10 repetitions. To perform the exercise, follow these steps:

1. Stand with both feet approximately shoulder width apart. Hold a barbell with your palms facing down (pronated grip).
2. Keeping your upper arms stationary, curl the weights up until the bar is at shoulder level.
3. Slowly return to the starting position.

Accuracy Counts!

The final component of injury free punching is target accuracy. For example, in a real world self-defense encounter you must avoid hitting hard body surfaces like the opponent's skull.

Believe it or not, many self-defense hand injuries are a result of striking the opponent's skull, which is extremely hard and resilient. It is likened to a crash helmet that protects the human brain from all forms of impact. I know several fighters who broke their hands when their fists accidentally connected with an opponent's forehead or skull.

Similarly, in double end bag training, you too must be careful where you place your punches. It's important that your strikes are accurate, and your punches are timed correctly. This can be especially challenging considering that the bag is always moving in unpredictable directions. Just keep in mind that one misplaced punch can easily injure your wrist.

Be Aware of What You Are Doing!

Learning how to punch correctly also means you will have to study and observe each and every punch in your arsenal and make certain they can handle the rigors of double end bag work. Through proper analytical observation, you can quickly identify the strengths and weaknesses of each punch in your arsenal. The best way to accomplish this is to methodically test each punch on the bag.

For example, take the most basic punch known to man - the rear cross. For those who may not be aware, the rear cross is one of the most effective punches in a fighter's arsenal.

Begin by standing approximately four to five feet from the bag. Then, assume a fighting stance with your left leg forward and your body positioned at a forty-five degree angle from the bag. Make certain both of your hands are properly clenched into fists and your head and chin are angled slightly down.

Now, deliver the punch, exhale and quickly twist and throw your rear arm and shoulder forward and towards the double end bag. Make certain to twist your rear leg, hip and shoulder forward and extend your rear arm straight. Do not lock out your rear arm when throwing the punch, be certain there is a slight bend in the elbow. Your punch should forcefully snap into the bag and then return to the starting position.

After delivering the punch to the bag, make the following important observations:

- What was the overall feeling of the punch when you delivered it? Did it feel rigid and forced or was it loose and fluid?
- What happened when your punch connected with the bag? Did the punch snap or crack the double end bag? Or did it just deflect to the side?

- Did anything feel strained or hurt when your fist initially connected with the bag?
- Was your punch accurate? Did you hit the bag exactly where you intended?
- Did you remember to exhale or did you hold your breath when you threw the punch?
- What happened to the structural integrity of your fist when you make contact with the punching bag? Did your fists open? Did your thumb get in the way? Did your wrist buckle inward?
- Which knuckle made initial contact with the bag?

You also might want to consider video taping yourself so you can quickly identify mistakes and errors in your punching form. Or perhaps you can have your training partner observe your punching technique and give you constructive feedback.

The Punching Mitts

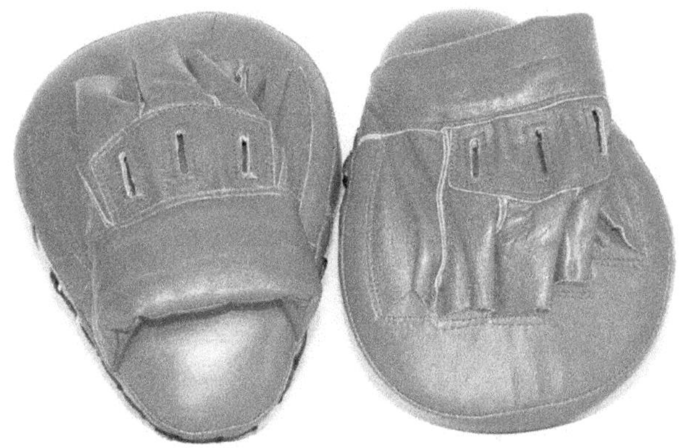

If you find the double end bag too frustrating to work with, you can always start off with the punching mitts (also called focus mitts) to examine your punching form.

Unlike the double end bag, the punching mitts don't move erratically are will allow you to progressively develop your punching form.

Punching mitts will challenge even the most seasoned fighter by improving both offensive and defensive fighting skills, punching speed, stamina, rhythm, endurance, accuracy, timing, reflexes, footwork, punching combinations, punching power and counter punching techniques.

The only downside to working with the punching mitts is they will require a training partner to hold them for you. The good news is, once you have trained on the mitts, you can then finally graduate to the double end bag.

Chapter 5
Double End Bag Techniques

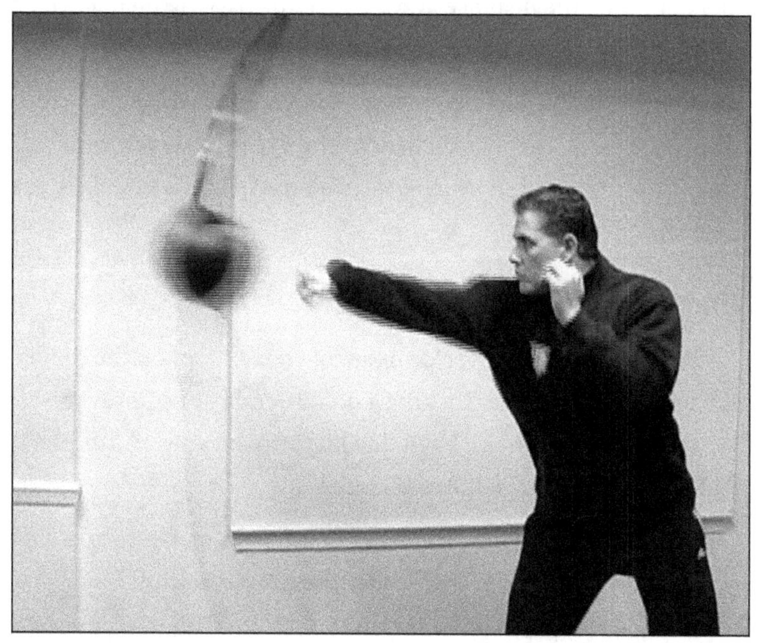

Angle and Distance Dictate the Strike

This chapter is going to focus on the different punches and strikes that can be performed on the double end bag. However, before we get into specific double end bag techniques, you'll first need to understand that the distance and angle of the bag will dictate which striking technique you can execute at any given moment.

Since the double end bag is suspended at approximately head level, we are going to focus on hand techniques. However, with regular training, you can also perform elbow strikes and well as head butt techniques.

What About Kicking the Bag?

While it's possible to perform kicking techniques on the double end bag, it's not practical. Kicking a double end bag requires you to perform high line kicks. High line kicks are kicking techniques directed to targets above the assailant's waist.

If you are training for reality-based self defense, never execute a high line kick in a fight. Here are just a few reasons why:

1. **Balance** - even the great kickers agree that high line kicks can cause them to lose their balance easily.
2. **Inefficiency** - they are not an efficient method of striking your assailant at this range.
3. **No power** - the less gravitational pull you put into a kick, the less power you will have.
4. **Clothing** - the clothing you are wearing can drastically limit your ability to execute a high line kick.
5. **Terrain** - you must have ideal terrain conditions to even consider throwing a high line kick.
6. **Flexibility** - exceptional flexibility is a prerequisite to execute

a high line kick properly.

7. **Appendage barriers** - high line kicks must generally be directed to the upper torso and head (why kick where the assailant's arms are?)
8. **Closest weapon to closest target rule** - your legs are closer to the assailant's low-line targets, not his high line targets.
9. **Interception** - high line kicks can be intercepted and grabbed by a well-seasoned fighter.
10. **Lack of speed** - high line kicks take longer to reach their target than low line kicks.
11. **Telegraphing** - due to the greater travel distance, high line kicks have a greater tendency to be telegraphed to the opponent.
12. **Distance from the ground** - high line kicks take your legs farther away from the ground, thus slowing down your overall compound attack.
13. **Energy expenditure** - high line kicks require more energy to execute than low-line kicks.
14. **Target exposure** - high line kicks unnecessarily expose several targets to the assailant during their delivery.
15. **High profile** - high line kicks are closer to the assailant's field of vision and are thus easier to see and to defend against.

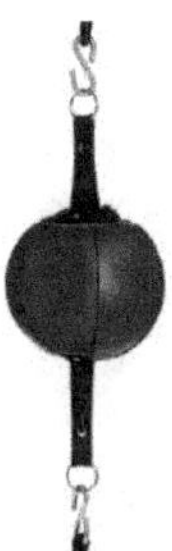

If you are going to execute kicking techniques in a real fight, always employ low line kicks to targets below the assailant's waist. They are efficient, effective, deceptive, non-telegraphic, and relatively safe. Low line kicking targets include the groin, quadriceps, common peroneal nerve (approximately 4 inches above the knee area), knee, and shin.

Punching Techniques

Punching techniques are the foundation of your double end bag training and they include the following:

- **Jab**
- **Rear cross (also called the straight right)**
- **Hook punch**
- **Uppercut punch**

The Jab

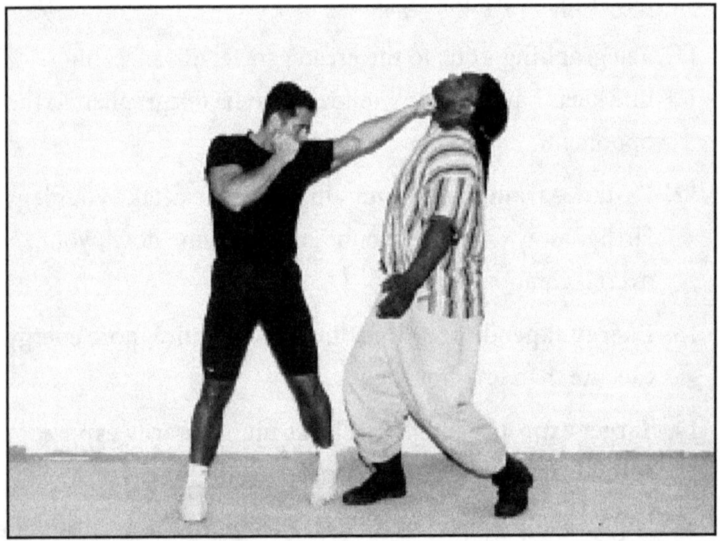

The jab is a foundation technique for boxers and mixed martial artists. This punch is thrown from your front hand and it has a quick snap when delivered.

1. Start off in a fighting stance with both of your hands held up in the guard position. Your fists should be lightly clenched with both of your elbows pointing to the ground.
2. To perform the punch, simultaneously step toward the bag and twist your front waist and shoulder forward as you snap

your front arm into the bag.

3. When delivering the punch, remember not to lock out your arm as this will have a "pushing effect" on the double end bag.
4. Quickly retract your arm back to the starting position.

One common mistake when throwing the jab is to let it deflect off to the side of the bag. Also, keep in mind that jabs can be delivered to the head (for a standard double end bag) or the body (if it's a double-double end bag).

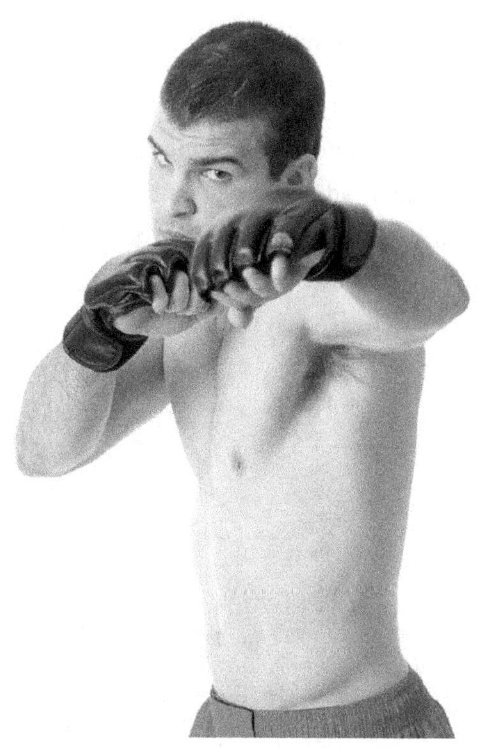

In boxing and mixed martial arts, the jab is an essential punch used to throw the opponent off balance, set him up for other blows, test his reflexes, and keep him from moving toward you.

Using the Jab for Street Self-Defense

While the jab might be appropriate for boxing, mixed martial arts and other forms of combat sport competition, it has no purpose in real world combat. The truth is the jab is combatively deficient for some of the following reasons:

- It lacks neutralizing power.
- It can expose you to a counter attack.
- It often agitates the assailant more than it harms him.
- It prolongs a self defense altercation and allows the assailant the opportunity to escalate his level of force against you.
- It's a probing and point scoring tool.

If self-defense is your interest and concern, you can simply replace the Jab with the Lead Straight punch. Like the jab, the lead straight is also a linear punch thrown from your lead arm, however this punch is much more powerful and can be used on the double end bag as well as real life self-defense situations.

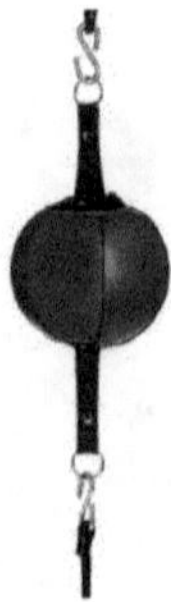

The lead straight is a linear punch thrown from your lead arm and contact is made with the center knuckle. To execute the lead straight, quickly twist your lead leg, hip, and shoulder forward. Snap your blow into the assailant's target and return back to the starting position. A common mistake is to throw the punch and let it deflect off to the side of the double end bag.

Rear Cross

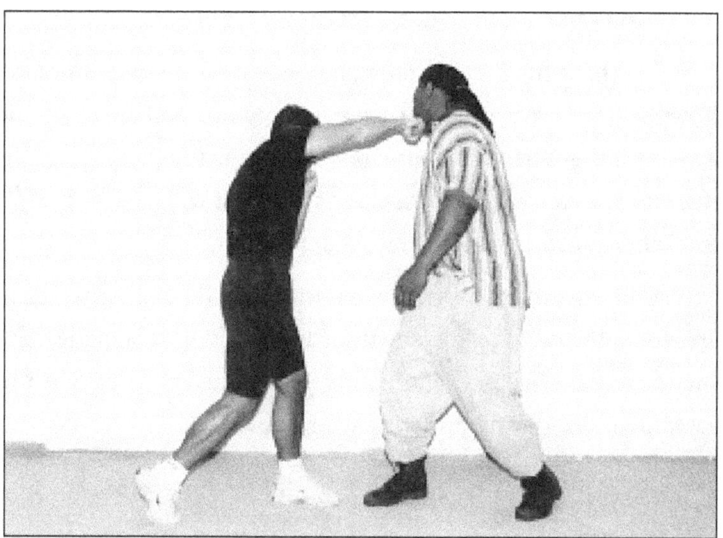

The rear cross (also called the straight right) is considered the heavy artillery of punches and it's thrown from your rear arm. To execute the punch, perform the following steps:

1. Start off in a fighting stance with both of your hands held up in the guard position. Your fists should be lightly clenched with both of your elbows pointing to the ground.
2. To perform the punch, quickly twist your rear hips and shoulders forward as you snap your rear arm into the double end bag. Proper waist twisting and weight transfer is of paramount importance to the rear cross. You must shift your weight from your rear foot to your lead leg as you throw the punch.
3. To maximize the impact of the punch, make certain that your fist is positioned horizontally. Avoid overextending the blow or exposing your chin during its execution.
4. Once again, do not lock out your arm when throwing the

punch. Let the power of the punch sink into the bag before you retract it back to the starting position.

When throwing the rear cross, be certain not to lock your elbow. Elbow locking is a common problem among novices. There should always be a slight bend in your elbow when the punch hits the bag. Remember, if your elbow locks upon impact, it will have a "pushing effect" and rob you of critical knock-out power.

Another common mistake when throwing the rear cross on the bag is to let the punch glide downwards after contact is made. Always remember, the trajectory of initiating your punch must also be the very same trajectory of retracting your punch.

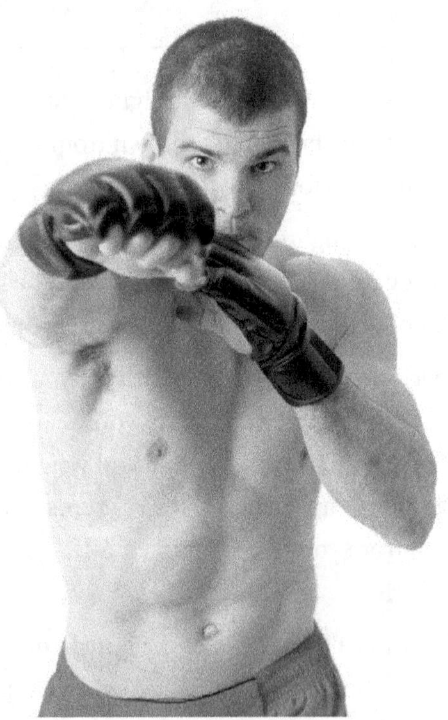

The rear cross is an extremely powerful punch that can be delivered effectively on the double end bag.

Hook Punch

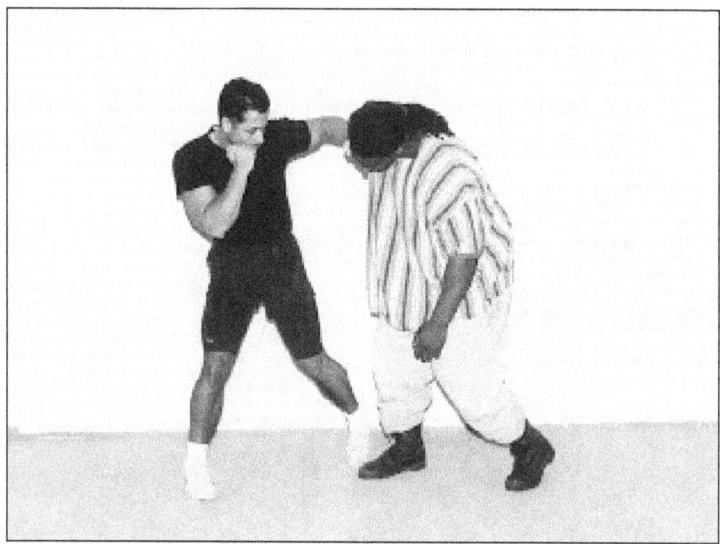

The hook is another devastating punch in your arsenal of techniques, yet it's also one of the most difficult to master. This punch can be performed from either your front or rear hand. There are actually two variations of the hook punch, they include:

- **Traditional Hook Punch**
- **Modified Hook Punch**

For the purposes of this book, I will teach you the traditional hook punch that is used in most boxing circles. Once again, if you would like to learn about the modified hook punch, which is used exclusively for street self-defense applications, you might want to look into my other books for more information.

1. Start in a fighting stance with your hand guard held up.
2. To execute the hook punch, quickly and smoothly, raise your elbow up so that your arm is parallel to the ground while simultaneously torquing your shoulder, hip, and foot into the direction of the blow.

3. When delivering the strike, be certain your arm is bent at least ninety degrees and that your wrist and forearm are kept straight throughout the movement.
4. As you throw the punch, your fist is positioned horizontally. The elbow should be locked when contact is made with the bag.
5. Return back to the starting position.

Uppercut Punch

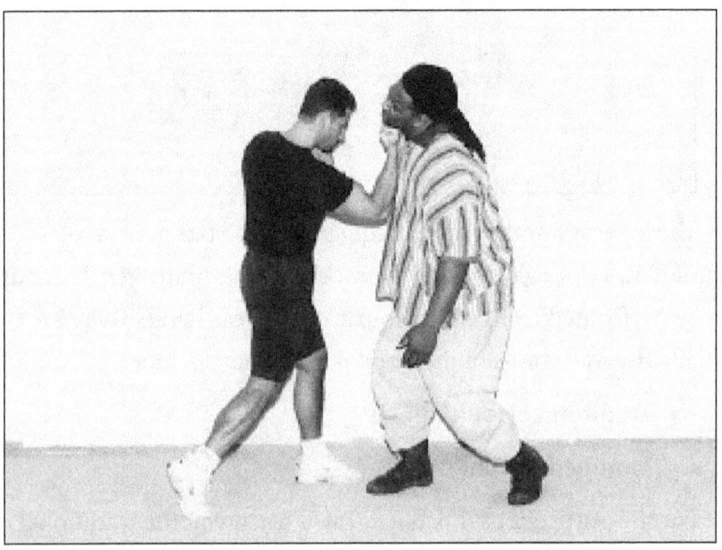

The uppercut is a another powerful punch that can be delivered from both the lead and rear arm. Due to its unusual angle of delivery, the uppercut is best practiced on either the punching mitts or uppercut bag. However, with a bit of careful practice it can be practiced on the double end bag.

1. Start off in a fighting stance with both of your hands held up in the guard position. Your fists should be lightly clenched with both of your elbows pointing to the ground.

2. To execute the uppercut, drop your shoulder and bend your knees.
3. Quickly, stand up and drive your fist upward and into the double end bag. Your palm should be facing you when contact is made with the bag. To avoid any possible injury, keep your wrists straight.
4. Make certain that the punch has a tight arc and that you avoid any and all "winding up" motions. A properly executed uppercut should be a tight punch and should feel like an explosive jolt.
5. Return back to the fighting stance.

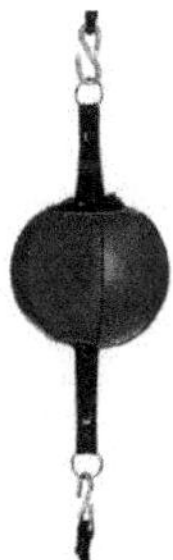

Remember to completely tighten your fists when impact is made with the double end bag. This action will allow your natural body weapon to travel with optimum speed and efficiency, and it will also augment the impact power of your punch.

Grappling Range

When it comes to double end bag training, grappling range striking techniques are going to appeal to three groups of people:

- **Self-defense practitioners**
- **Mixed martial artists (MMA)**
- **Martial artists (traditional and eclectics)**

You can add a couple grappling range strikes to your double end bag workouts. Here are two:

- **Elbow strikes**
- **Short arc hammer fist strikes**

Horizontal Elbow

The elbows are devastating weapons that can be used in the grappling range. They are explosive, deceptive and very difficult to stop. Elbows can generally be delivered horizontally, vertically, diagonally and they can be thrown from either your front or rear arm.

Let's just take a look at the body mechanics of the horizontal elbow strike

1. Start off in a fighting stance with both of your hands held up in the guard position. Make certain that you are standing in close proximity to the bag.
2. To execute the elbow strike, quickly and smoothly, raise your elbow up so that your arm is parallel to the ground.
3. Next, simultaneously torquing your shoulder, hip, and foot into the direction of the bag. The tip of your elbow should make contact with the target.
4. Return back to the starting position.

Diagonal Elbow (traveling downward)

The diagonal elbow strike travels diagonally downward to the double end bag. It can be delivered from either the right or left side of the body. To execute the strike, perform the following:

1. Start off in a fighting stance with both of your hands held up in the guard position. Make certain that you are standing in close proximity to the bag.
2. To execute the elbow strike, rotate your elbow back, up, and over while quickly whipping it downward to your desired target.
3. Bend your knees as your body descends with the strike. Your palm should be facing away from you when making contact.
4. The striking surface is the elbow point.
5. Return back to the starting position.

Vertical Elbow

The vertical elbow travels vertically to the double end bag and it can be executed from either the right or left side of the body. To perform the strike, do the following:

1. Start off in a fighting stance with both of your hands held up in the guard position. Make certain that you are standing in close proximity to the bag.
2. To execute the elbow strike, raise your elbow vertically (with the elbow flexed) until your hand is next to the side of your head. The striking surface is the point of the elbow.
3. The power for this strike is acquired through the quick extension of the legs at the moment of impact with the target.
4. Return back to the starting position.

Short Arc Hammer Fist

The short arc hammer fist is a quick and powerful strike that is delivered at close range. To deliver the hammer fist, perform the following steps:

1. Start off in a fighting stance with both of your hands held up in the guard position. Make certain that you are standing in close proximity to the bag.
2. Begin by raising your fist with your elbow flexed. Quickly whip your clenched fist down in a vertical line onto the double end bag. Remember to keep your elbow bent on impact and maintain your balance throughout execution of the movement.
3. Return back to the starting position.

Chapter 6
Workout Routines

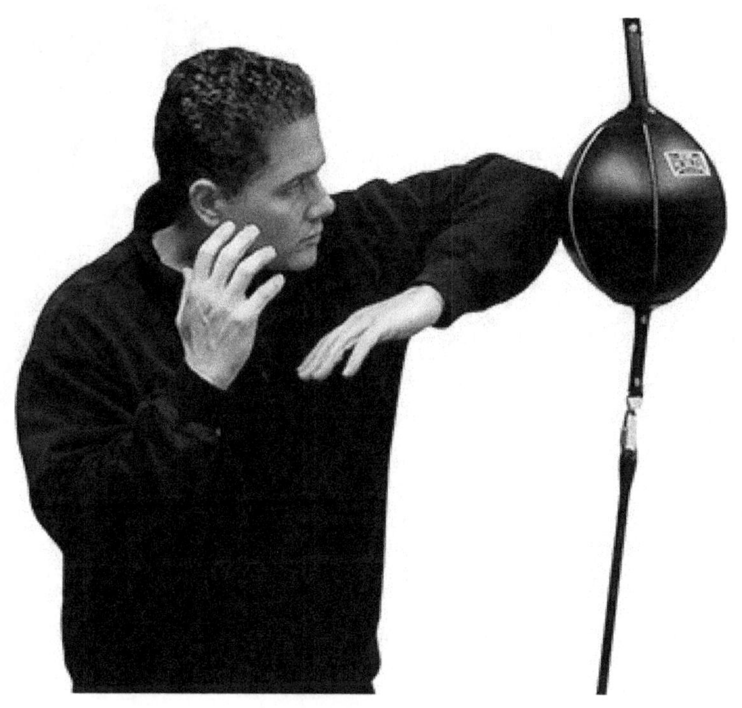

The Three Training Methodologies

Before introducing you to the different double end bag routines featured in this chapter, it's important to first discuss the three training methodologies.

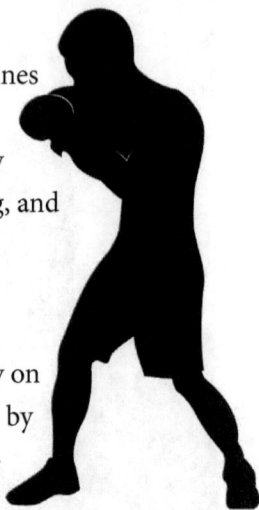

Essentially, all of the double end bag routines presented in this book will fall under one of three different types of training methods; they are proficiency training, conditioning training, and street training. Let's take a look at each one.

Conditioning Training

Conditioning Training focuses exclusively on "time-based" workouts and it's primarily used by boxers, mixed martial artists, kickboxers, self-defense technicians, and fitness enthusiasts who wish to train on the double end bag for specified period of time called *rounds*. Depending on the practitioner's level of conditioning, each round can range anywhere from one to five minutes. Each round is then separated by either 30-second, one-minute or two-minute breaks. A good double end bag workout consists of at least five to eight rounds.

Conditioning Training is performed at a moderate pace, and it develops cardiovascular fitness, muscular endurance, fluidity, rhythm,

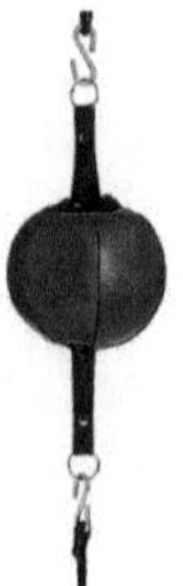

Conditioning training can also be used when sparring, shadow boxing, working on the heavy bag, skipping rope, and focus mitt training.

distancing, timing, speed, footwork, and balance. Many fitness enthusiasts who are looking to burn fat will use this methodology as it tends to burn a significant amount of calories.

Conditioning Training does require that you have a fundamental understanding of combining punches and kicks together into logical combinations.

As I discussed in some of my other books, a combination or *compound attack* is the logical sequence of two or more techniques thrown in strategic succession. For example, a jab followed by a rear cross is considered to be a basic punching combination.

Proficiency Training

The second training methodology is Proficiency Training and it's generally used by martial artists and self-defense practitioners who want to sharpen one specific punch, kick, or strike at a time by executing it over and over for a prescribed number of repetitions. Each time the technique is performed with "clean" form at various speeds. Punches are also carried out with the eyes closed to develop a kinesthetic "feel" for the action.

Proficiency Training on the double end bag develops speed, accuracy, non-telegraphic movement, balance, and psychomotor skill.

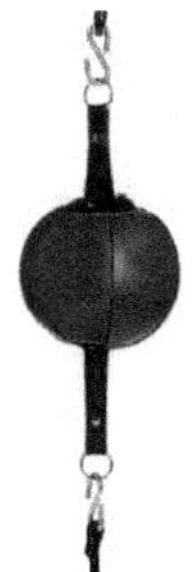

Proficiency training is not just limited to martial arts and self-defense. It can also been used by boxers who want to develop and sharpen a specific punching technique. For example, a boxing coach might have his student jab at the bag for a specific amount of repetitions.

Street Training

The third and final training methodology is Street Training, and it's specially designed for reality-based self-defense preparation.

Since most self-defense altercations are explosive, lasting an average of 20 seconds, the practitioner must prepare for this possible scenario. This means delivering explosive and powerful compound attacks with vicious intent for approximately 20 seconds, resting one minute, and then repeating the process. Well-conditioned athletes can go longer. In fact, a few of my students are capable of performing the street training methodology uninterrupted for a full minute.

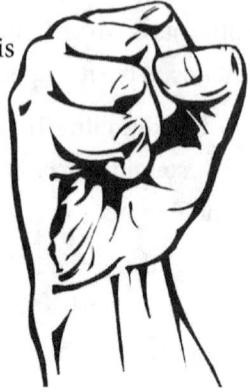

Street Training prepares you for the stress and immediate fatigue of a real fight. It also develops speed, power, explosiveness, target selection and recognition, timing, footwork, pacing, and breath control. You can also practice this methodology in different lighting, on different terrains, and in various environmental settings.

Street Training is not just limited to double end bag training. For example, you can prepare yourself for multiple assailants by having your training partners attack you with focus mitts from a variety of angles, ranges, and target postures. For 20 seconds, go after them with vicious and powerful offensive techniques.

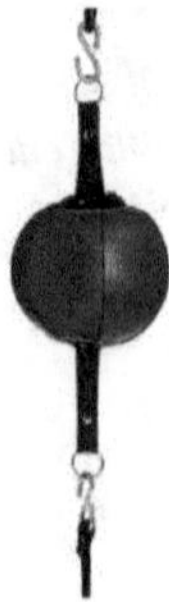

Street training is predicated on explosiveness. The offensive techniques that barrage the bag should possess a sudden and immediate outburst of violent energy. Your attack should never be progressive in nature; it does not build in speed and power. It begins and ends explosively.

Technique Always Comes First!

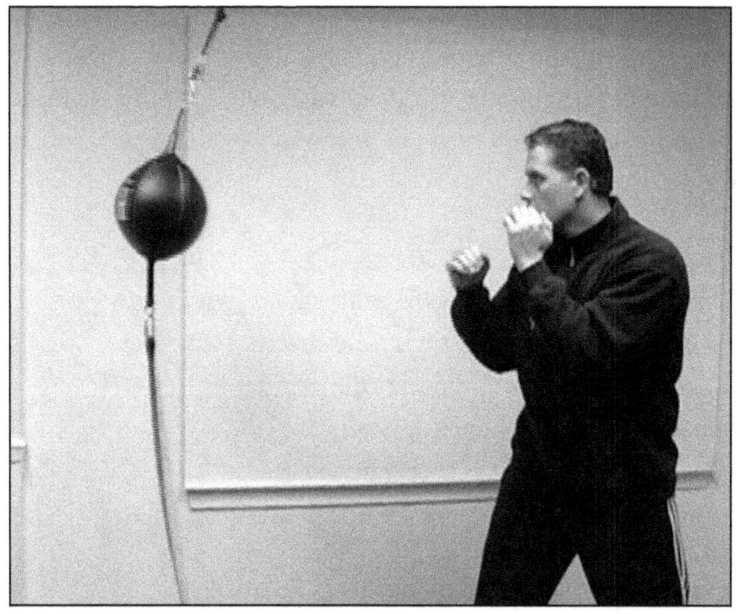

Take your time when working out on the double end bag. If you are learning how to use it for the very first time, I strongly urge you to take your time and develop the proper punching mechanics before tearing into the bag.

Remember, the double end bag is a serious piece of training equipment, and if you're not careful you can get injured when using it. Double end bag training is also demanding on the body. Avoid premature exhaustion by pacing yourself during your workouts. Remember, it's not a race! Enjoy the process of learning how to use the bag with skill and finesse.

Get a Check-Up First

Double end bag training can be very taxing on your heart. So, before you begin any exercise program, including those suggested in this book, it is important to check with your doctor to see if you have any condition that might be aggravated by this type of strenuous exercise.

Warming Up

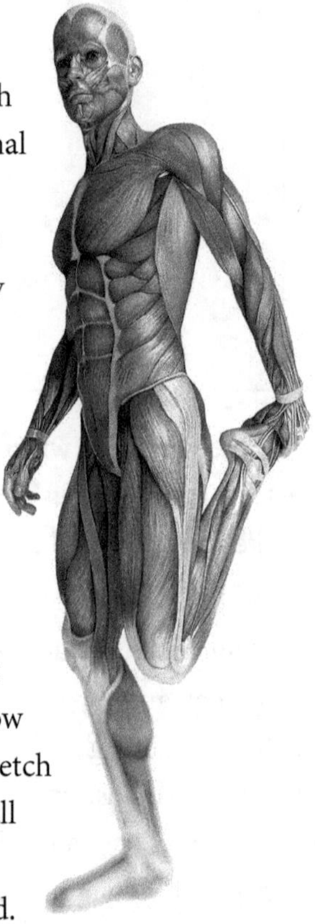

Before beginning any of the drills, it's important that you first warm up and stretch out. Warming up slowly increases the internal temperature of your body while stretching improves your workout performance, keeps you flexible, and helps reduce the possibility of an injury.

Some of the best exercises for warming up are jumping jacks, rope skipping or a short jog before training. Another effective method of warming up your muscles is to perform light and easy movements with the weights.

When stretching out, keep in mind that all movements should be performed in a slow and controlled manner. Try to hold your stretch for a minimum of sixty seconds and avoid all bouncing movements. You should feel mild tension on the muscle that is being stretched. Remember to stay relaxed and focus on what you are doing. Here are seven stretches to get you started.

- **Neck stretch** - from a comfortable standing position, slowly tilt your head to the right side of your neck, holding it for a count of twenty. Then tilt your head to the left side for approximately twenty seconds. Stretch each side of the neck at least three times.

- **Triceps stretch** - from a standing position, keep your knees slightly bent, extend your right arm overhead, hold the elbow of your right arm with your left hand, and slowly pull your right elbow to the left. Keep your hips straight as you stretch your triceps gently for thirty seconds. Repeat this stretch for the other arm.
- **Hamstring stretch** - from a seated position on the floor, extend your right leg in front of you with your toe pointing to the ceiling. Place the sole of your left foot in the inside of your extended leg. Gently lean forward at the hips and stretch out the hamstrings of your right leg. Hold this position for a minimum of sixty seconds. Switch legs and repeat the stretch.
- **Spinal twist** - from a seated position on the floor, extend your right leg in front of you. Raise your left leg and place it on the outside of your right leg. Place your right elbow on the outside of your left thigh. Stabilize your stretch with your elbow and twist your upper body and head to your left side. Breathe naturally and hold this stretch for a minimum of thirty seconds. Switch legs and repeat this stretch for the other side.

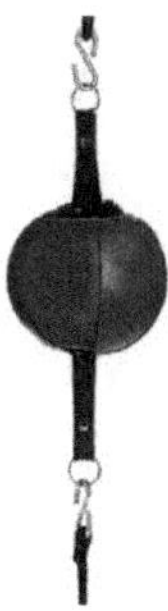

You need a good stretching program designed to loosen up every muscle group. Remember, you can't punch, or otherwise execute the necessary body mechanics if you're "tight" or inflexible. Stretching on a regular basis will also increase the muscles' range of motion, improve circulation, reduce the possibility of injury, and relieve daily stress.

- **Quad stretch** - assume a sitting position on the floor with your hamstrings folded and resting on top of your calves. Your toes should be pointed behind you, and your instep should be flush with the ground. Sit comfortably into the stretch and hold for a minimum of sixty seconds.
- **Prone stretch** - lay on the ground with your back to the floor. Exhale as you straighten your arms and legs. Your fingers and toes should be stretching in opposite directions. Hold this stretch for thirty seconds.
- **Groin stretch** - sit on the ground with the soles of your feet touching each other. Grab hold of your feet and slowly pull yourself forward until mild tension is felt in your groin region. Hold this position for a minimum of sixty seconds.

Avoiding Overtraining & Burnout

Burnout is defined as a negative emotional state acquired by physical overtraining. Some symptoms of burnout include physical illness, boredom, anxiety, disinterest in training, and general sluggish behavior. Whether you are a beginner or expert, you're susceptible to burnout. Here are a few suggestions to help avoid burnout in your training:

1. Make your workouts intense but enjoyable.
2. Vary your training routine (i.e., hard day/easy day routine).
3. Train to different types of music.
4. Pace yourself during your workouts - don't try to do it all in one day.
5. Listen to your body- if you don't feel up to training, skip a day. Missing a day or two won't kill you.
6. Work out in different types of environments.
7. Use different types of training equipment.

8. Work out with different training partners.
9. Keep accurate records of your training routine.
10. Vary the intensity of your training throughout your workout.

What's Next?

Finally, it's time to take a look at the different types of double end bag workouts. I'll start with a beginner drill to get you started.

Beginner Exercise
Open Hand Tap Drill

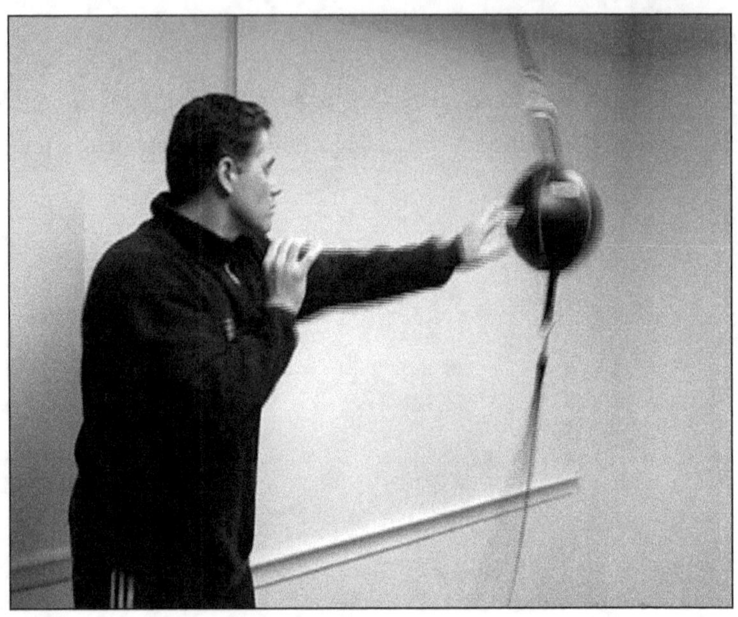

The first exercise I'm going to show you is called the open hand tap drill. This is a beginner exercise that's designed to get you comfortable with making contact with the bag. (If you do have experience working on the double end bag, feel free to skip this exercise.)

To begin, the drill perform the following steps:

1. Start off in a fighting stance with both of your hands held up in the guard position. Make certain that you are standing approximately arms reach from the bag.
2. Open both of your hands with your fingers in a semi-clawed position.
3. Next, reach out with your front arm and tap the bag with

your palm. As the bag returns, reach out with your rear arm and tap the bag again.

4. Alternate tapping the double end bag for a period of 30 seconds.
5. Remember to perform this drill is a controlled rhythmic manner.

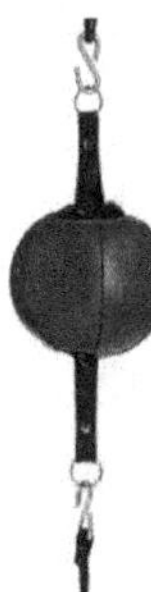

If you discover that it's too difficult to alternate arms in this drill, you can perform it with one arm at a time.

Open Hand Tap Drill Demonstration

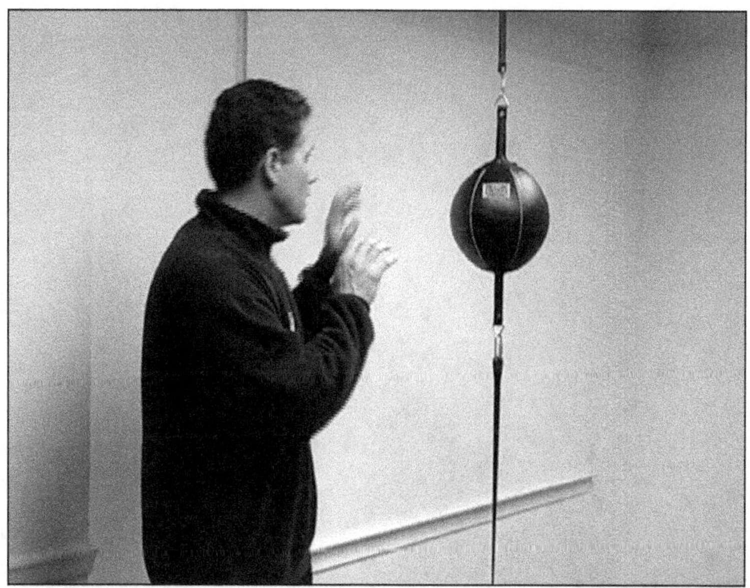

Step 1: Assume a fighting stance and open your hands with your fingers in a semi-clawed position.

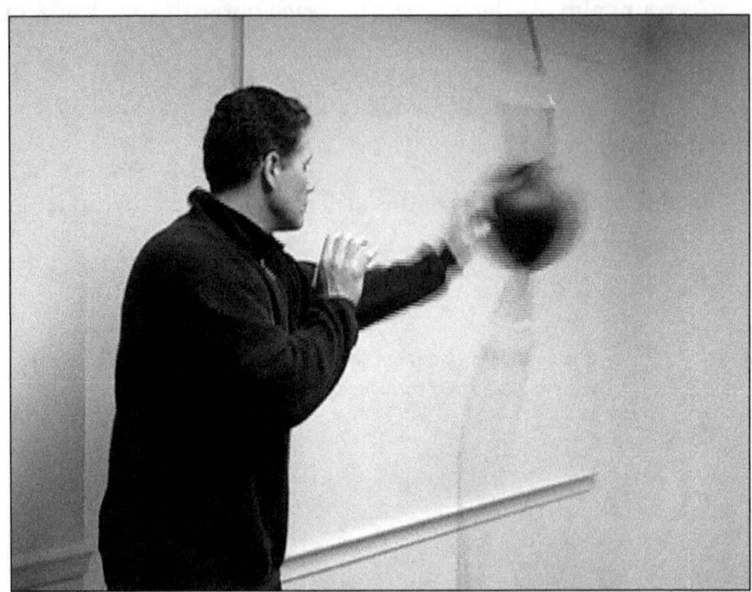

Step 2: Reach out with your front hand and tap the double end bag with your palm.

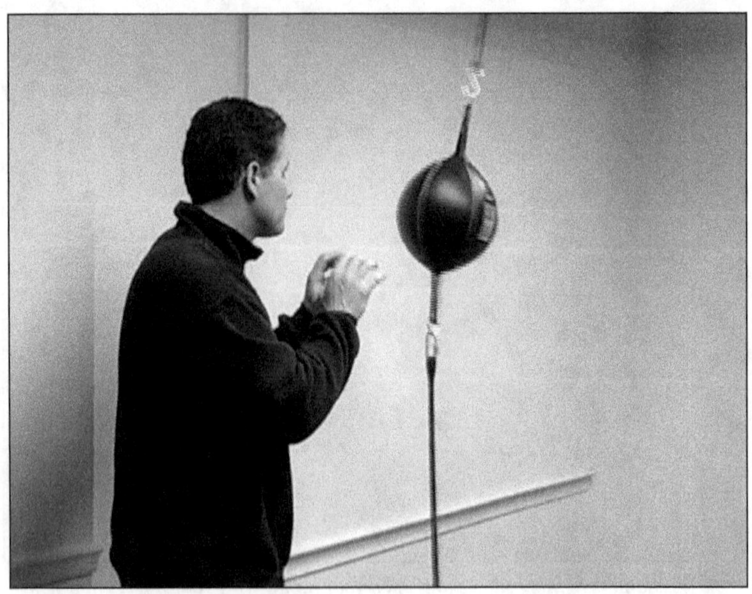

Step 3: Quickly retract your lead arm from the bag.

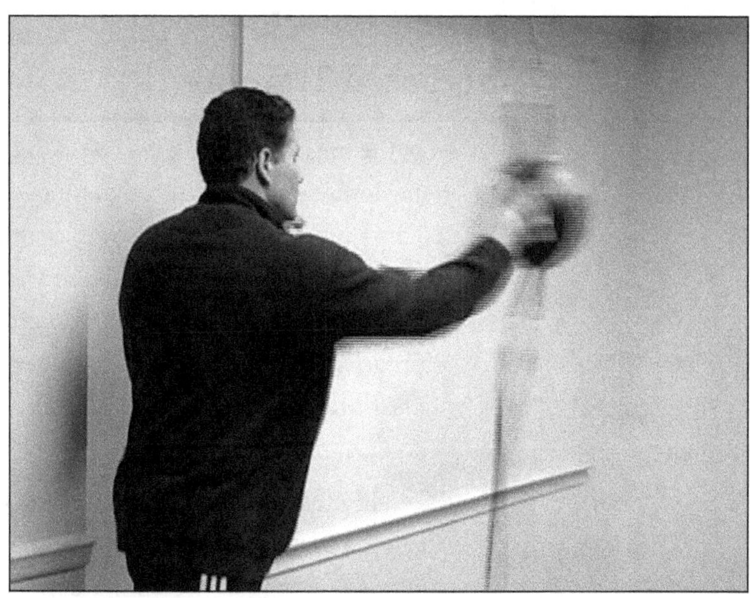

Step 4: Next, reach our with your rear arm and tap the bag again.

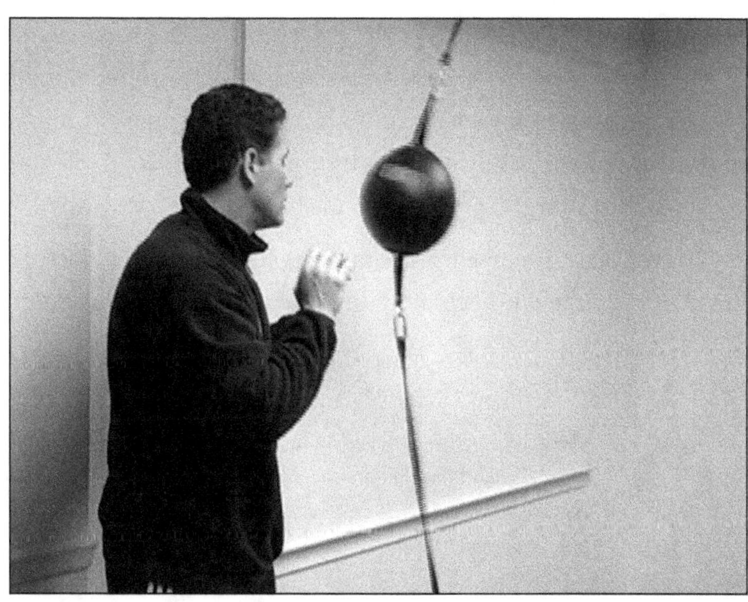

Step 5: Return to the starting position.

Workout Routine #1
Time-Based Training

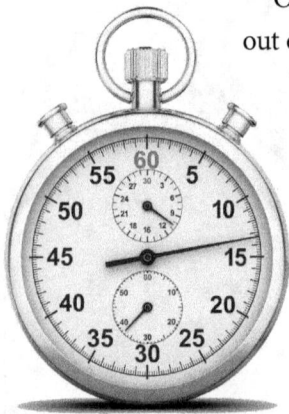

One of the most popular ways of working out on the double end bag is through time-based training. A time-based double end bag workout is based on rounds, and it's an ideal way to structure your workout program. Before you begin, decide on the duration of your rounds as well as the rest intervals.

In most cases, mixed martial artists, boxers and kick boxers will work the double end bag for three-minute rounds with one-minute rest periods. Depending on their level of conditioning and specific training goals, they might do this for a total of 5 to 10 rounds.

Initially, you'll need to experiment with both the round duration and rest intervals to see what works best for you. Remember to start off slow and progressively build up the intensity and length of your workouts. Don't forget to work with the bag and not try to kill it!

To get you started, here are some sample time-based workouts you might want to try. Keep in mind, the Advanced Level workouts

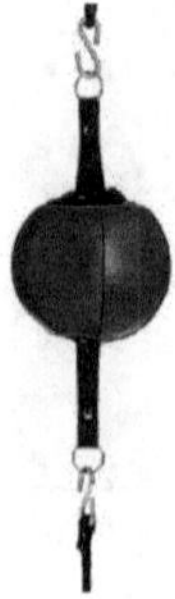

Besides the actual body mechanics of punching, there are several other elements that comprise a punching combination. They include attack rhythms, height variations, the cadence of delivery, and practitioner movement.

are for elite fighters who have a minimum of 5 years of double end bag training and conditioning.

Time-Based Double End Bag Workouts

Skill Level	Duration of Each Round	Rest Period	Total Number of rounds
Beginner	1 minute	2 minutes	3
Beginner	1 minute	1 minute	3
Beginner	2 minutes	2 minutes	3
Beginner	2 minutes	1 minute	3
Intermediate	3 minutes	2 minutes	5
Intermediate	3 minutes	1 minute	5
Intermediate	3 minutes	2 minutes	6
Intermediate	3 minutes	1 minute	6
Advanced	4 minutes	2 minutes	8
Advanced	4 minutes	1 minute	8
Advanced	5 minutes	2 minutes	10
Advanced	5 minutes	1 minute	10

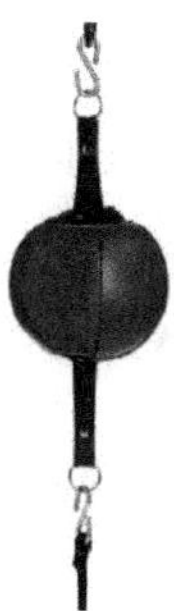

All time-based workouts will require you to invest in a workout timer. Luckily, there are dozens of smartphone apps that mimic the same features of an actual interval timer. These workout apps are convenient, inexpensive and can be found at your favorite online app store.

What Combinations Should I Throw?

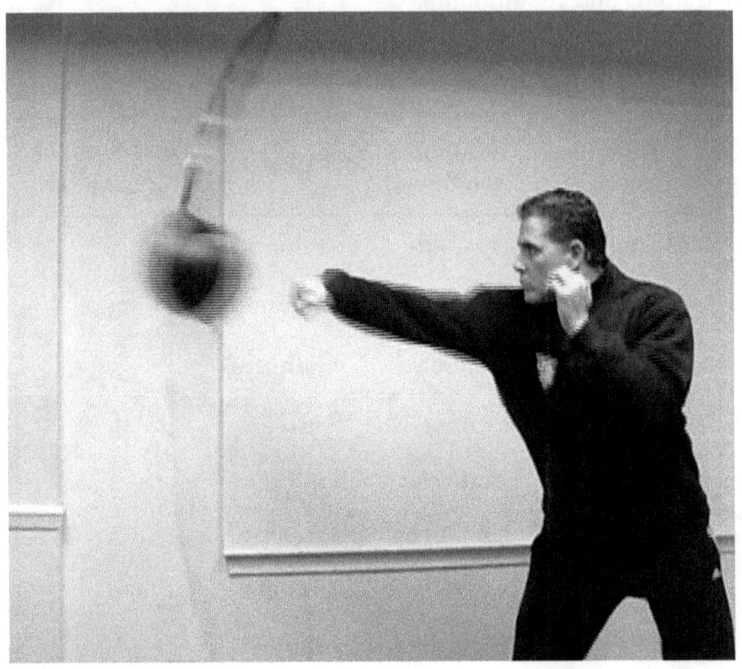

What follows are just a few punching combinations you can perform during your time-based workouts.

Once again, this book assumes you can perform the basic punching skills, including the jab, rear cross, hook, and uppercut. However, if you are not familiar with these foundational techniques, please see the step-by-step instructions featured in the previous chapter of this book.

When reading the combination sequence on the following pages, please note the word *high* indicates punches delivered at head level when using a standard double end bag, while *low* represents punches delivered to the lower bag when using a double-double end bag or a Mexican style double end bag.

Combinations for the standard double end bag

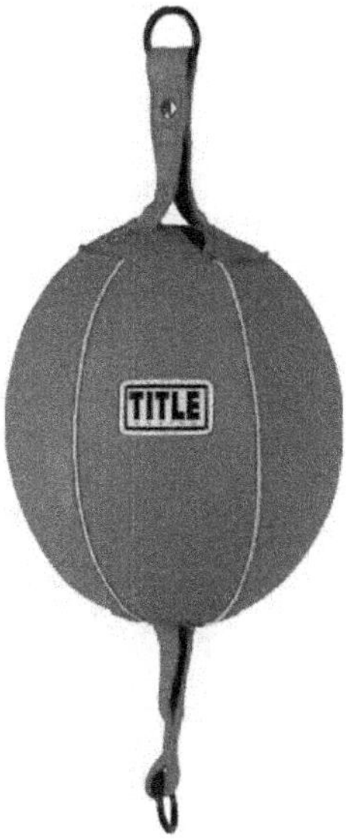

- Jab - Jab
- Jab - Jab - Rear Cross
- Jab - Rear Cross
- Jab - Rear Cross - Jab
- Jab - Rear Cross - Jab - Rear Cross
- Jab - Jab - Rear Cross - Jab
- Jab - Jab - Rear Cross - Lead Hook
- Jab - Jab - Rear Cross - Lead Uppercut
- Jab - Rear Cross - Jab
- Jab - Rear Cross - Lead Hook
- Jab - Rear Cross - Lead Hook - Rear Hook
- Jab - Rear Cross - Lead Hook - Rear Hook - Lead Uppercut
- Jab - Rear Hook
- Jab - Lead Hook
- Jab - Lead Hook - Rear hook
- Rear Cross - Lead Hook
- Rear Cross - Lead Hook -Rear Cross
- Rear Cross - Lead Hook - Lead Hook - Rear Hook
- Rear Cross - Lead Uppercut -Rear Cross - Lead Hook

The standard double end bag.

- Rear Cross - Lead Hook - Rear Cross - Lead Hook - Rear Hook
- Lead Hook - Rear Hook
- Lead Hook - Rear Hook - Lead Hook
- Jab - Rear Cross - Lead Hook - Rear Uppercut
- Rear Uppercut - Lead Hook
- Rear Uppercut - Lead Hook - Rear Hook
- Rear Uppercut - Lead Uppercut
- Lead Uppercut - Rear Uppercut
- Rear Uppercut - Lead Uppercut - Rear Uppercut

Combinations for a double-double end bag or Mexican style double end bag

- Jab (low) - Jab (low)
- Jab (high) - Jab (low)
- Jab (low) - Jab (high)
- Jab (high) - Jab (high) - Rear Cross (low)
- Jab - Rear Cross (low)
- Jab - Rear Cross (low) - Jab
- Jab - Rear Cross - Lead Hook (low) Jab - Rear Cross - Lead Hook (low) - Rear Hook (low)
- Jab - Rear Cross - Lead Hook (high) -

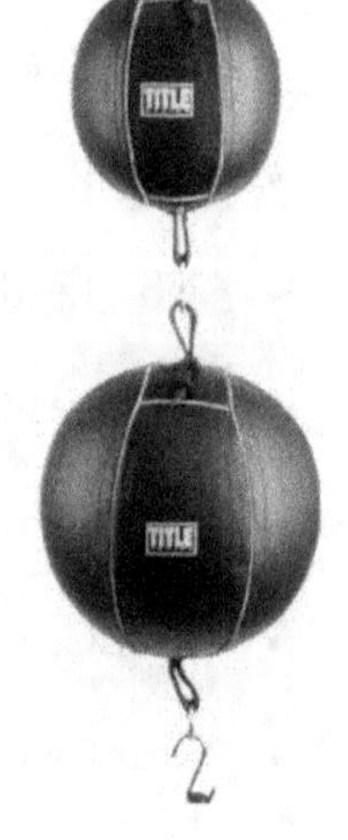

The double-double end bag.

Rear Hook (low)

- Jab - Rear Cross - Lead Hook (low) - Rear Hook (high)
- Jab - Rear Hook (low)
- Jab - Lead Hook (low)
- Jab - Lead Hook (low) - Rear hook (low)
- Jab - Lead Hook (high) - Rear hook (low)
- Jab - Lead Hook (low) - Rear hook (high)
- Jab - Jab - Rear Cross - Lead Hook (low)
- Jab - Rear Cross - Lead Hook (high) - Rear Hook (low) - Lead Uppercut

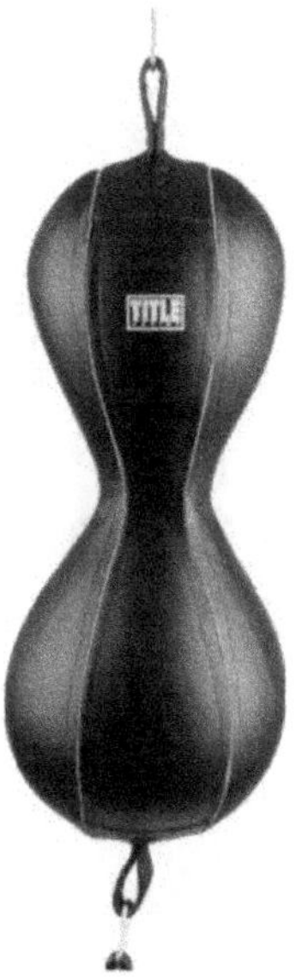

The Mexican style double end bag.

- Rear Cross - Lead Hook - Lead Hook - Rear Hook (low-high-high-low)
- Rear Cross - Lead Hook - Lead Hook - Rear Hook (high-low-low-high)
- Rear Cross - Lead Hook - Rear Cross - Lead Hook - Rear Hook (high-high-low-high-low)
- Rear Uppercut - Lead Hook (low)
- Rear Uppercut - Lead Hook (low) - Rear Hook (low)
- Rear Uppercut - Lead Hook (high) - Rear Hook (low)

Take a Look!

On the following pages, you'll be able to see some of these combinations put into action.

Combination #1: jab-jab (double jab)

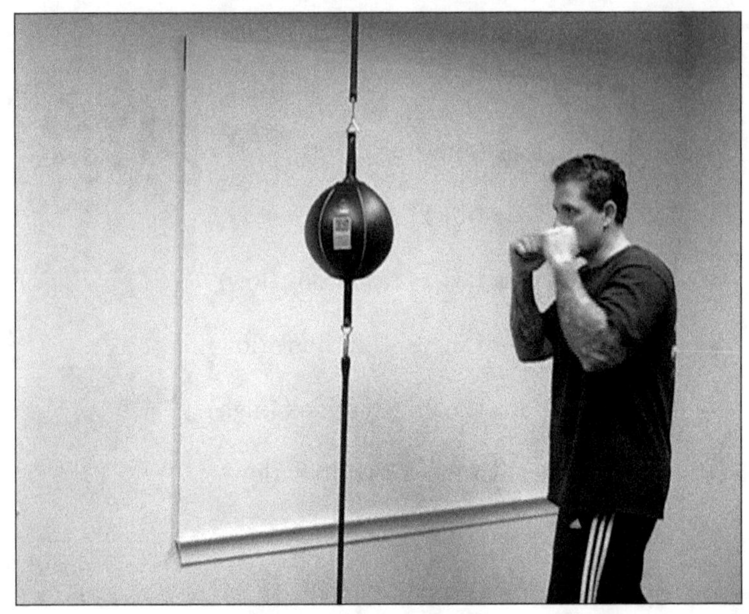

Step 1: Begin from a fighting stance.

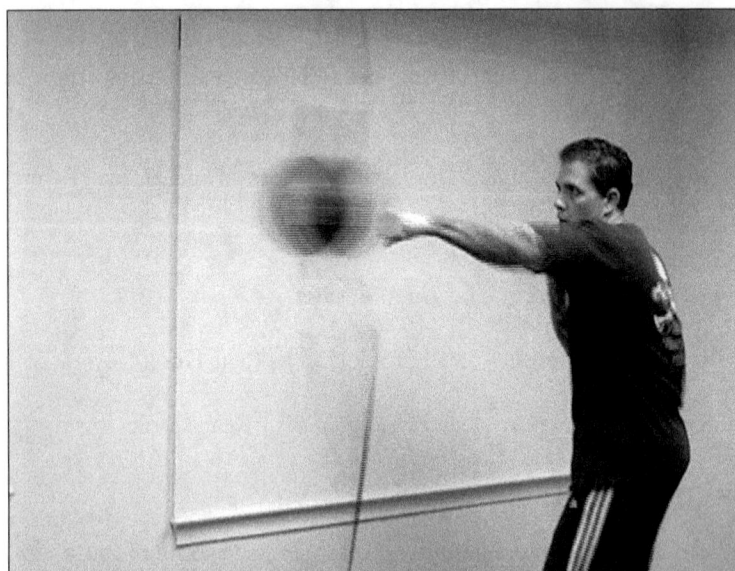

Step 2: Extend your lead arm forward and jab the bag.

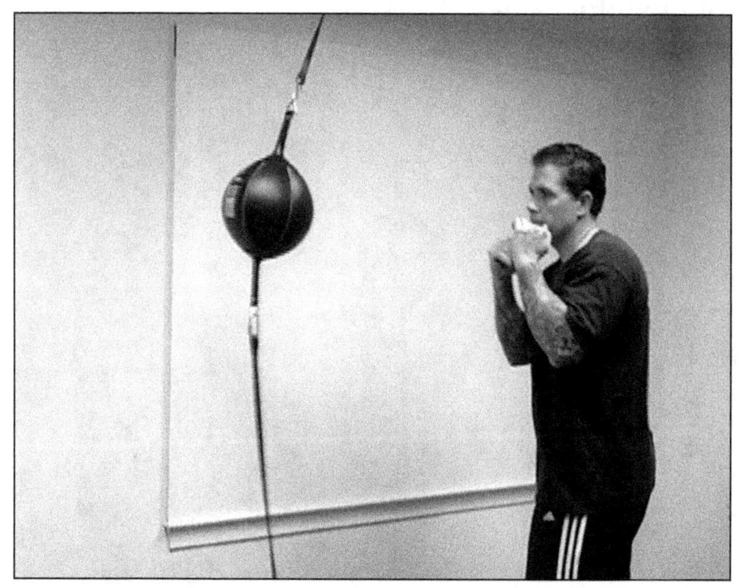

Step 3: Return to the stance position.

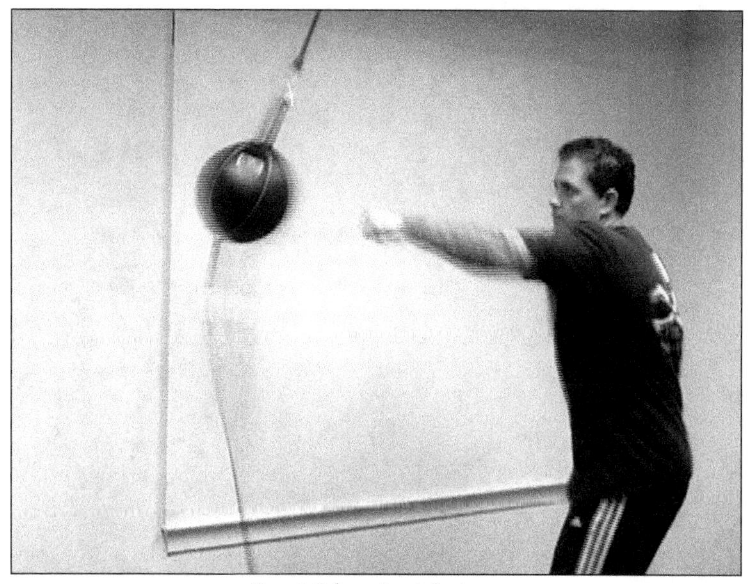

Step 4: Jab again at the bag.

Combination #2: jab-rear cross

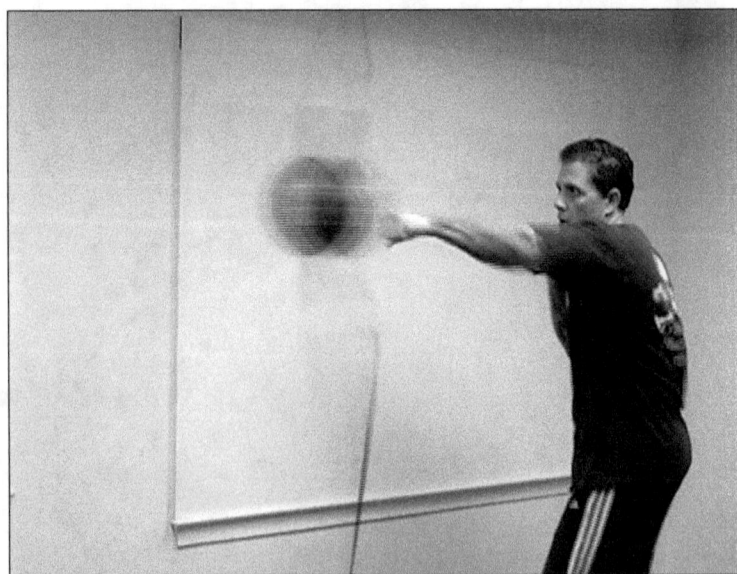

Step 1: Begin from a fighting stance.

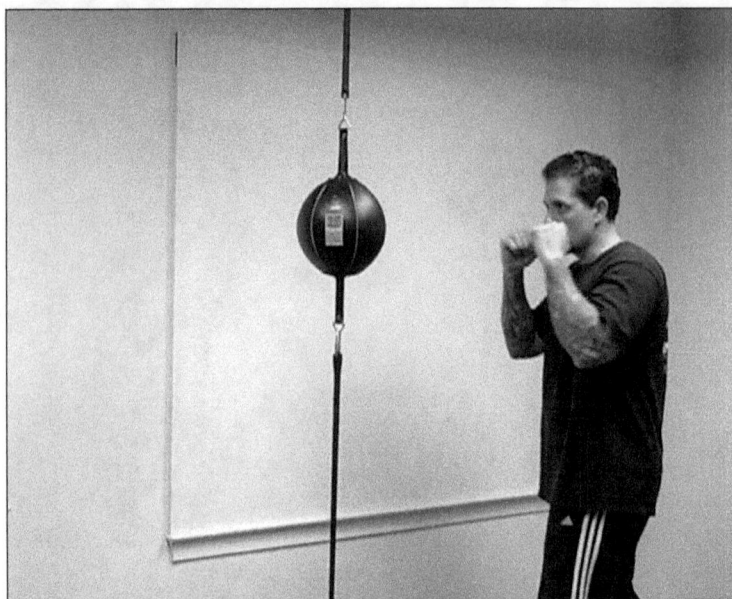

Step 2: Jab the double end bag.

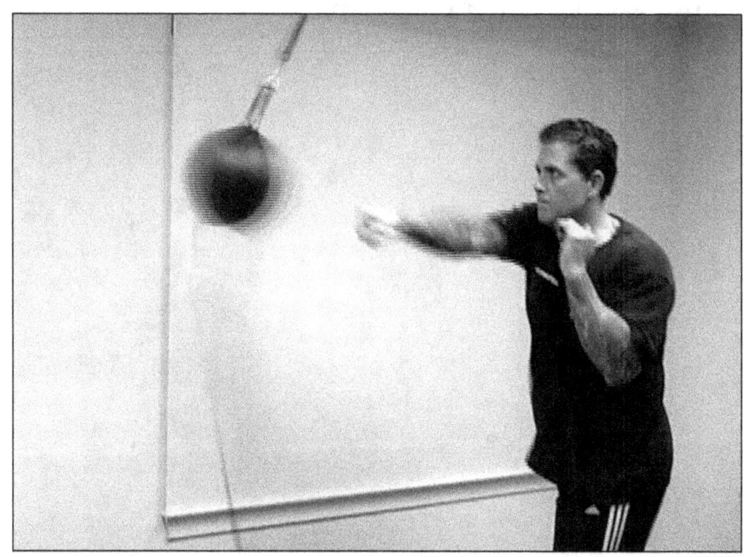

Step 3: Next, deliver a rear cross.

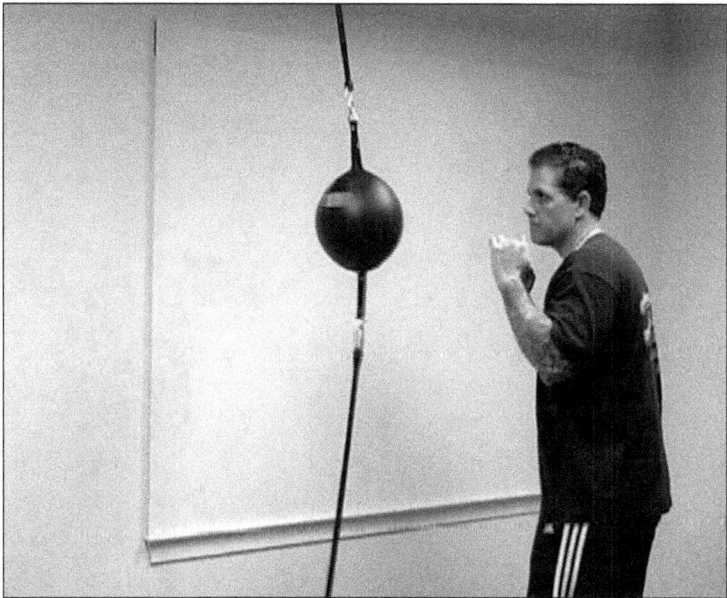

Step 4: Return to the stance position

Combination #3: rear cross-jab

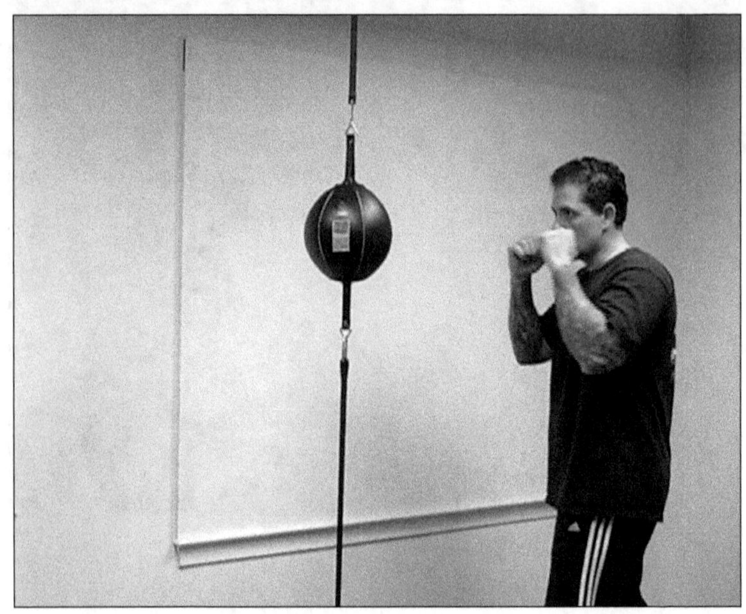

Step 1: Begin from a fighting stance.

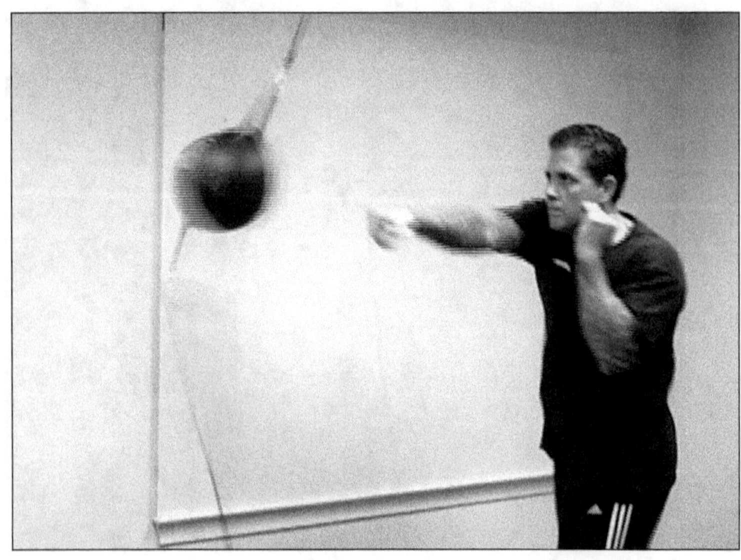

Step 2: Deliver a rear cross.

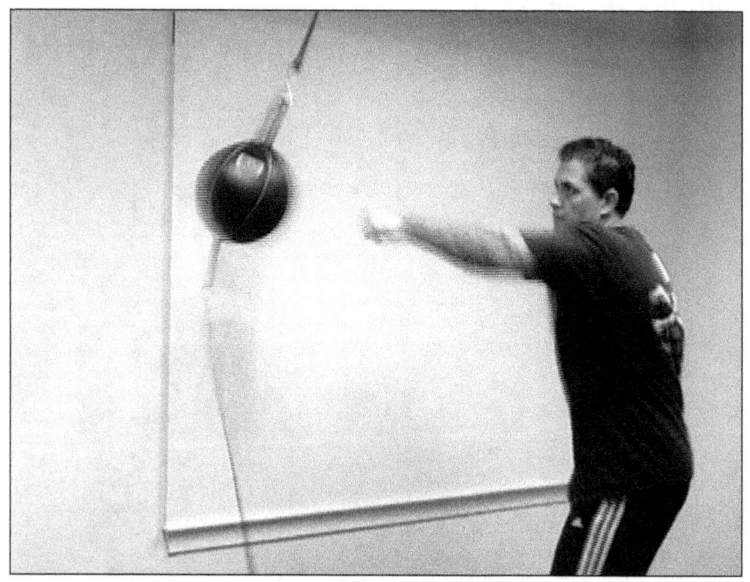

Step 3: Next, jab again at the bag.

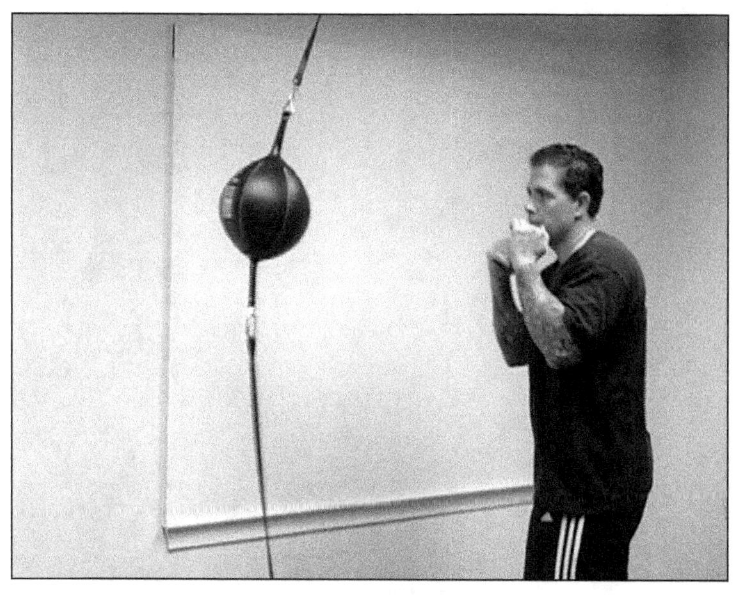

Step 4: Return to the stance position.

Combination #4: jab-rear cross-rear cross

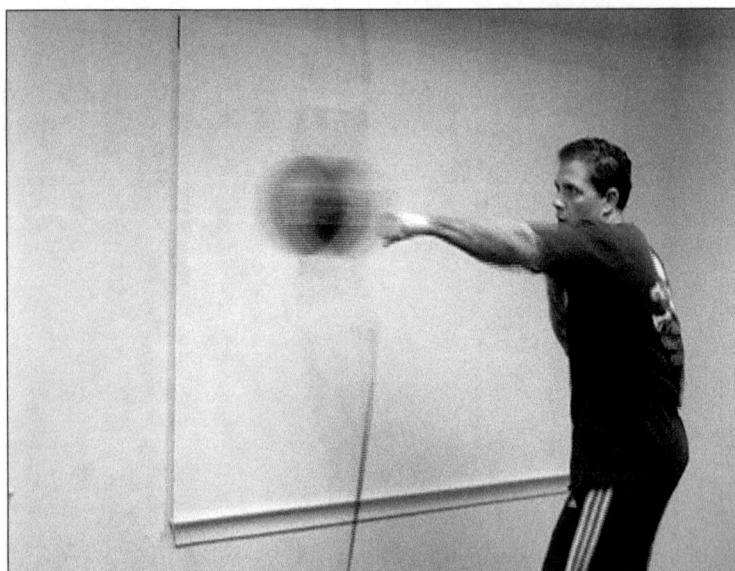

Step 1: Begin from a fighting stance.

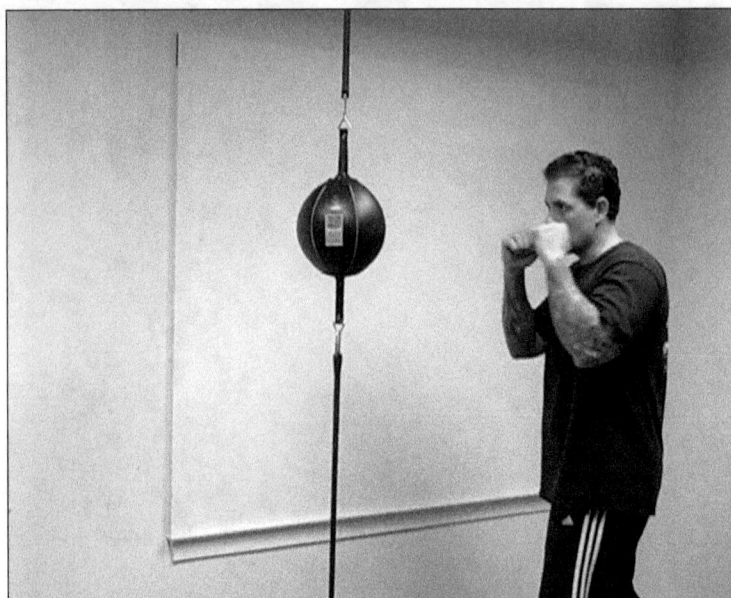

Step 2: Jab the double end bag.

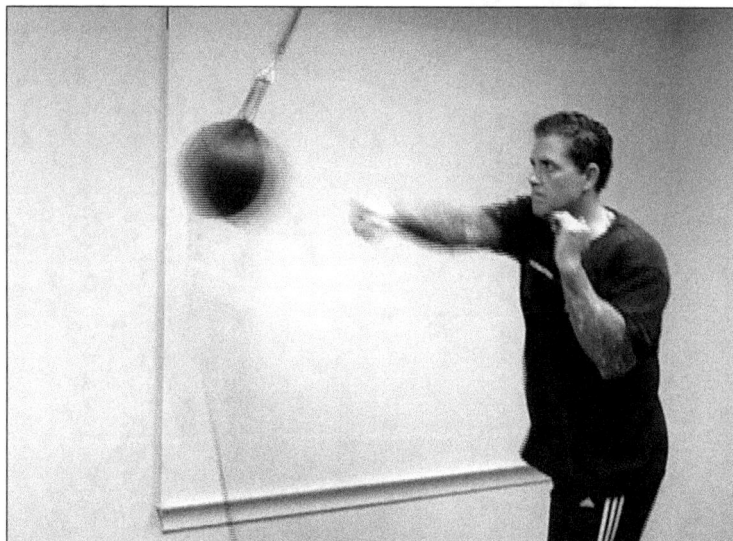

Step 3: Next, deliver a rear cross.

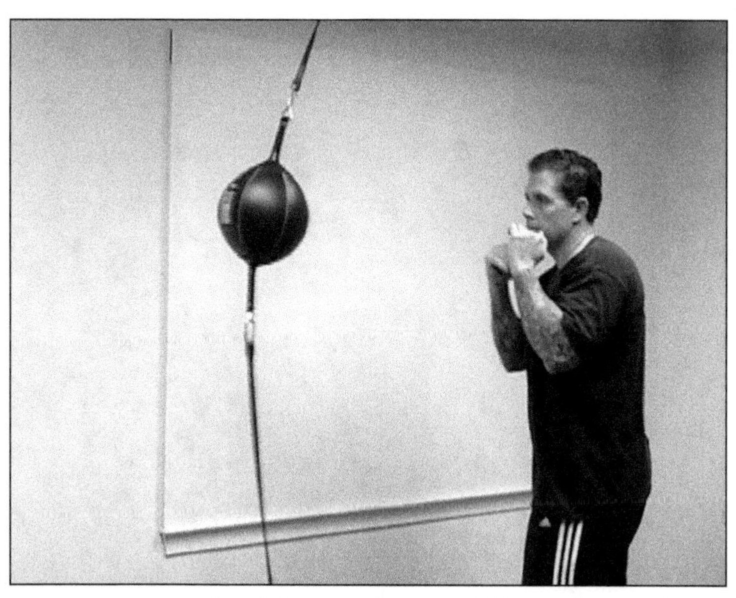

Step 4: Return to the stance position.

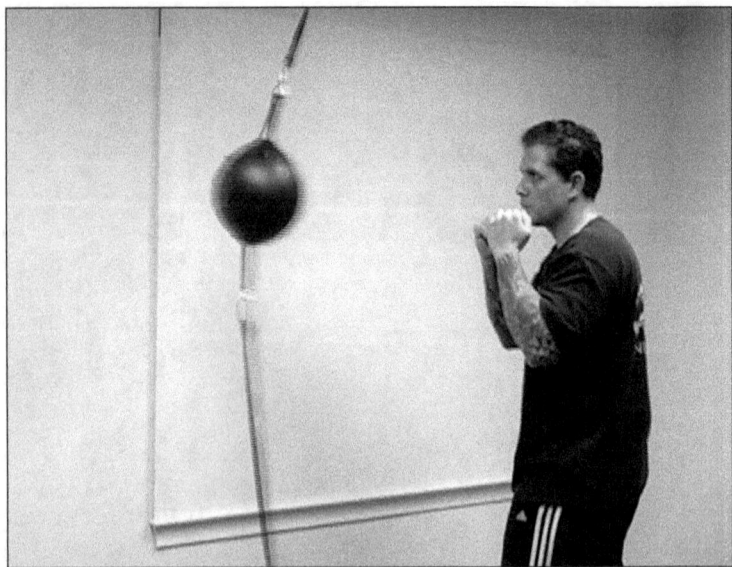

Step 5: Deliver another rear cross.

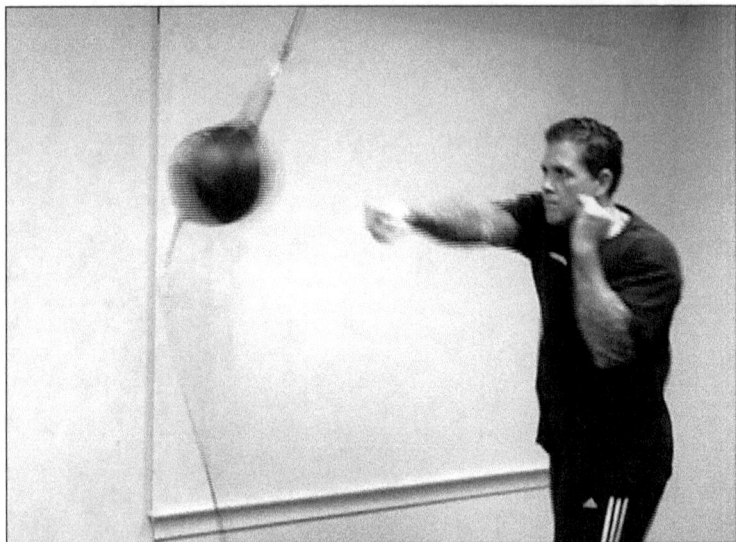

Step 6: Return to your stance.

Combination #5: jab-rear cross-hook-hook

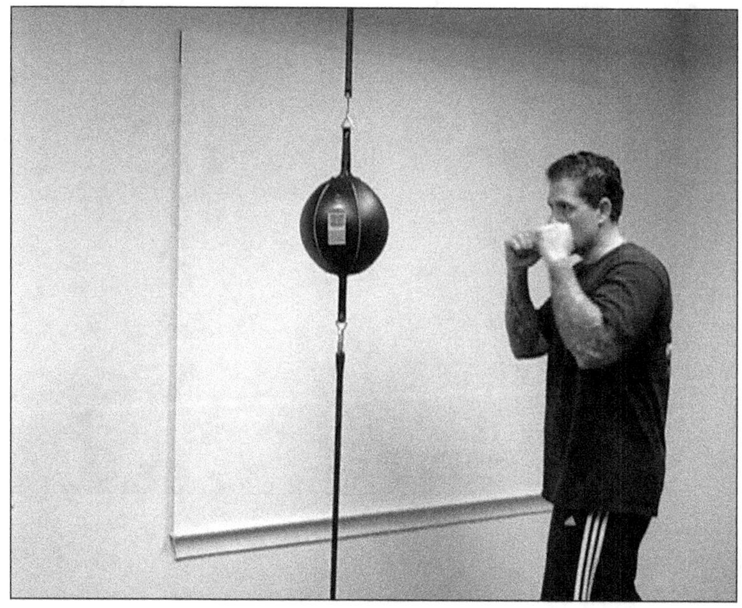

Step 1: Begin from a fighting stance.

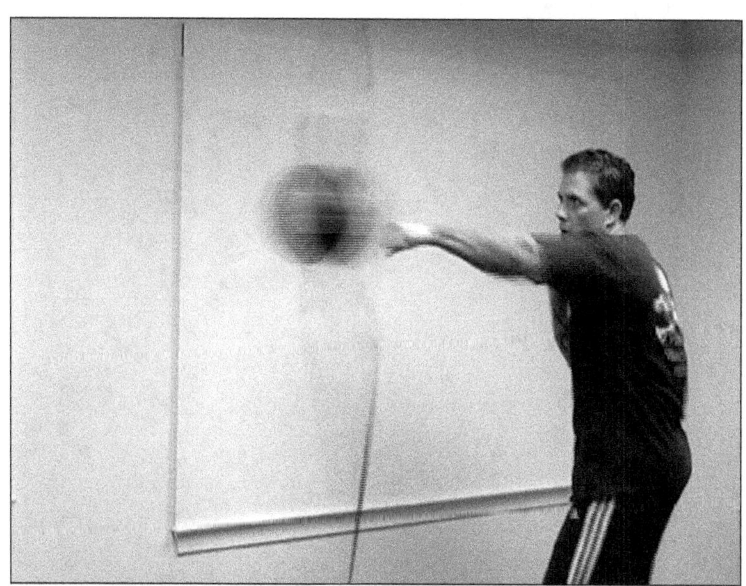

Step 2: Extend your lead arm forward and jab the bag.

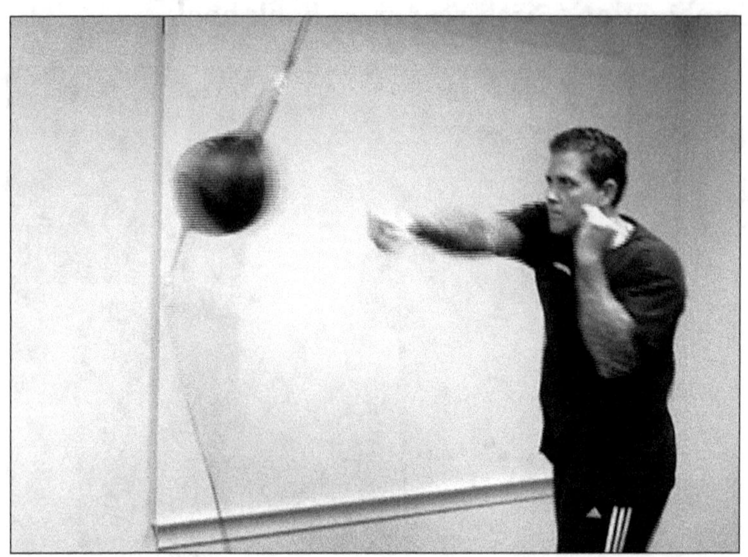

Step 3: Deliver a rear cross.

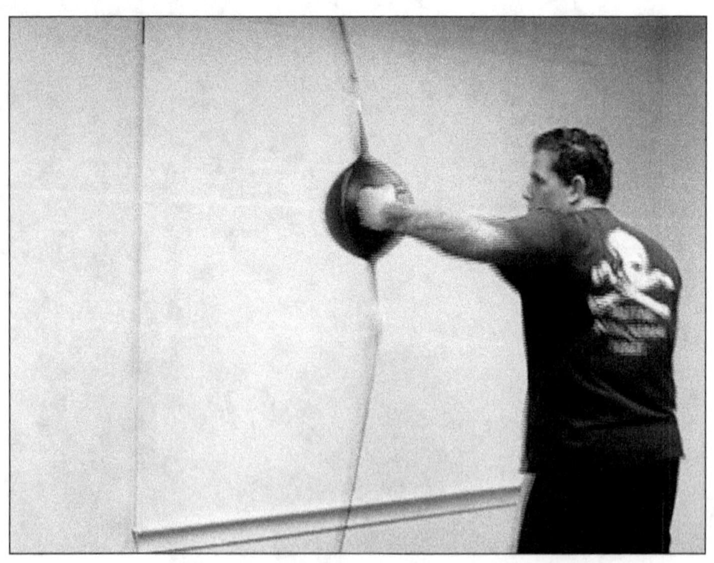

Step 4: Immediately follow with a lead hook punch.

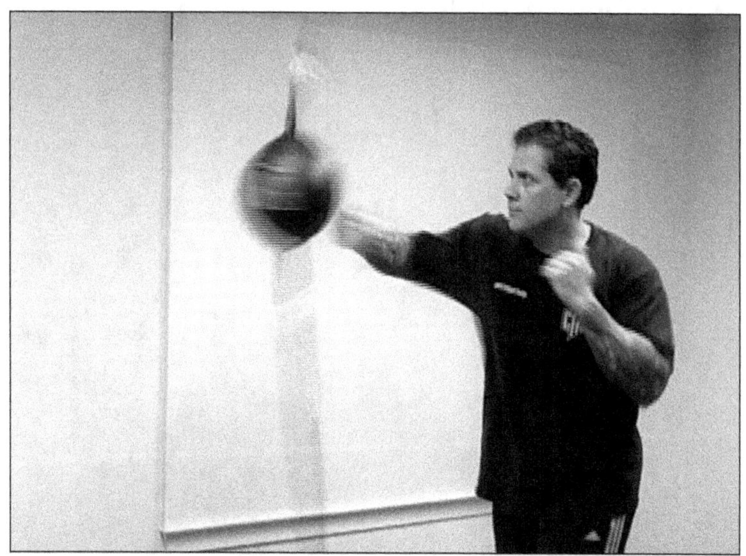

Step 5: Next, deliver a rear hook.

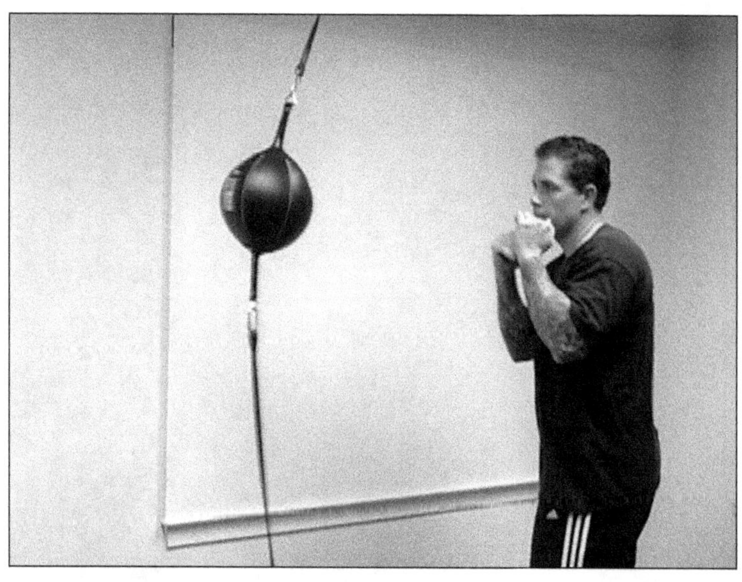

Step 6: Return to your stance.

Combination #6: jab-lead hook-rear cross

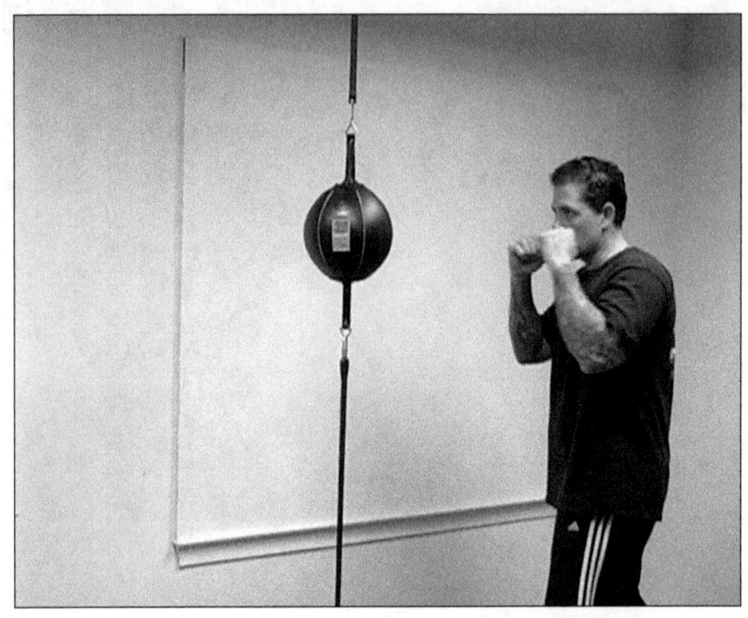

Step 1: Begin from a fighting stance.

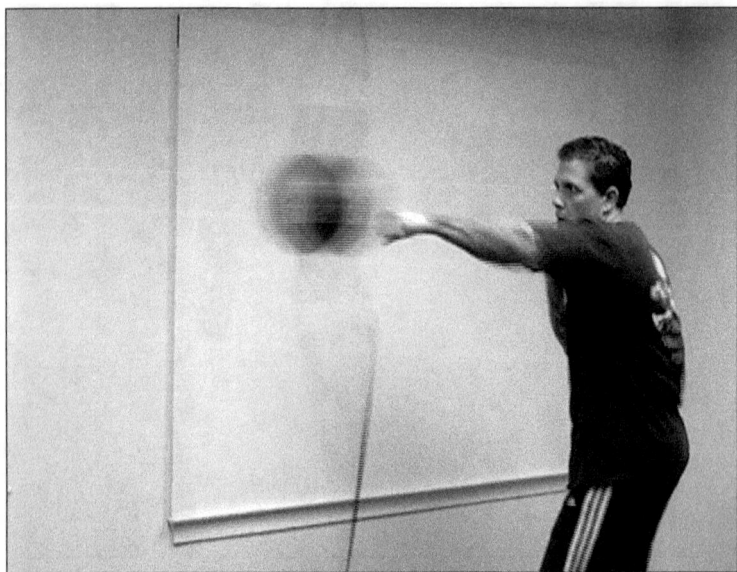

Step 2: Jab the double end bag.

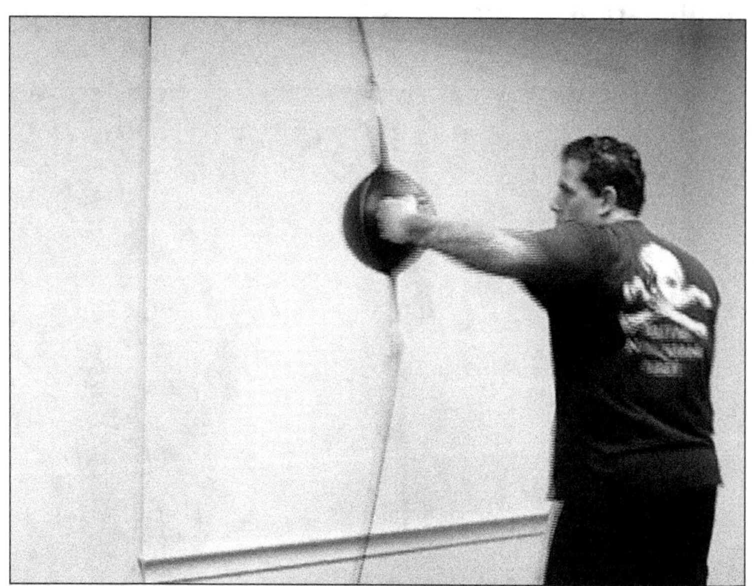

Step 3: From the same arm, deliver a lead hook.

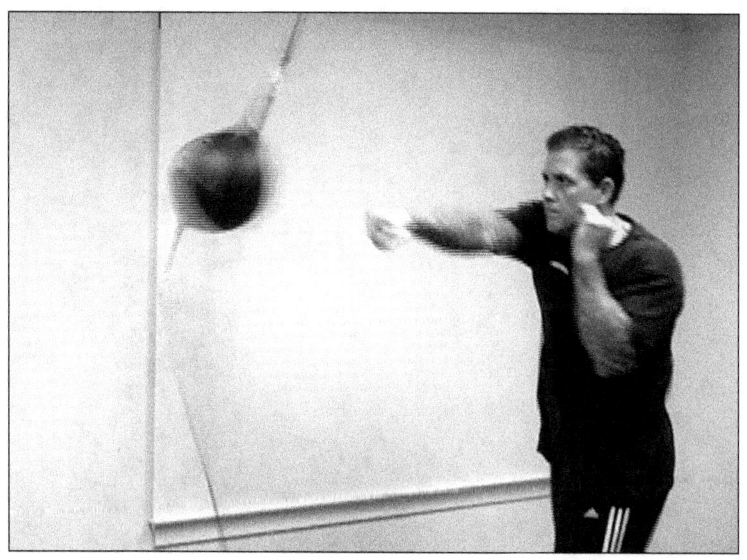

Step 4: Next, throw a rear cross.

Combination #7: rear cross-lead hook-lead hook-rear hook

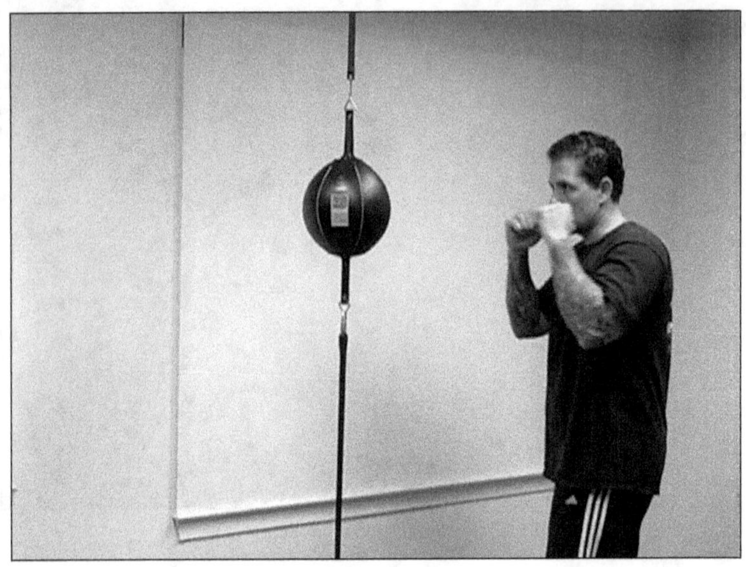

Step 1: Begin from a fighting stance.

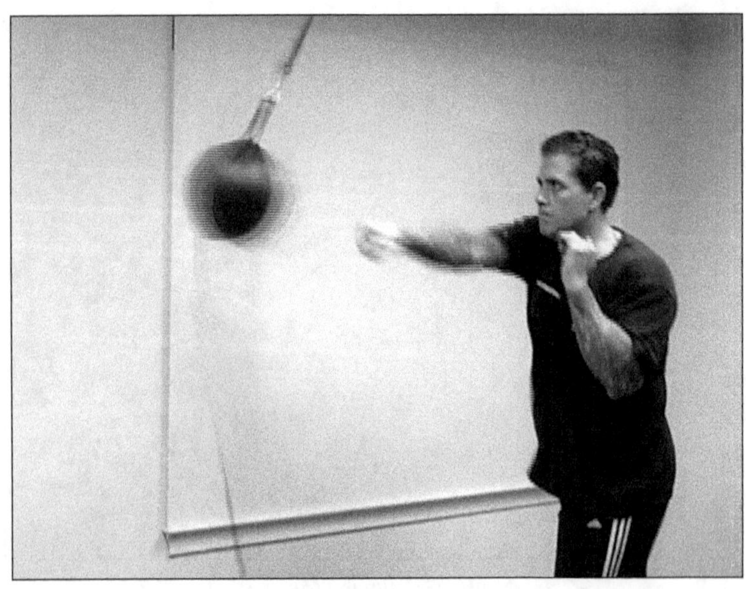

Step 2: Deliver a rear cross at the bag.

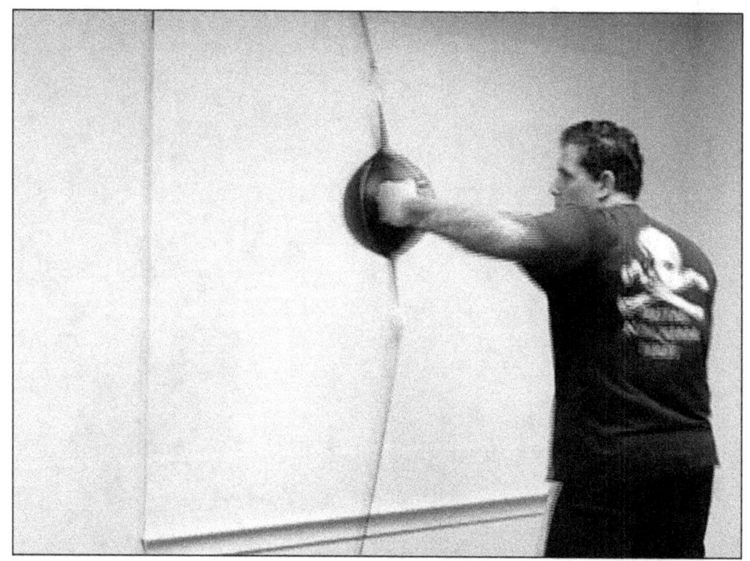

Step 3: Next, a lead hook.

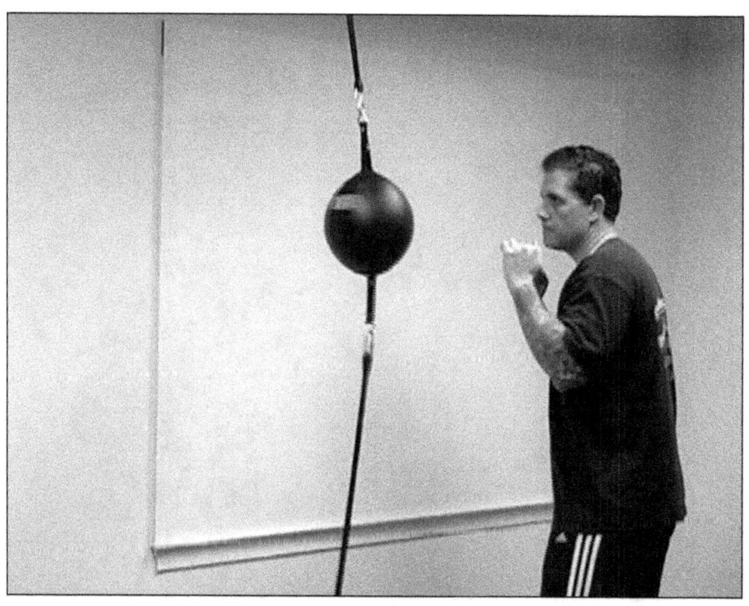

Step 4: Quickly retract your punch.

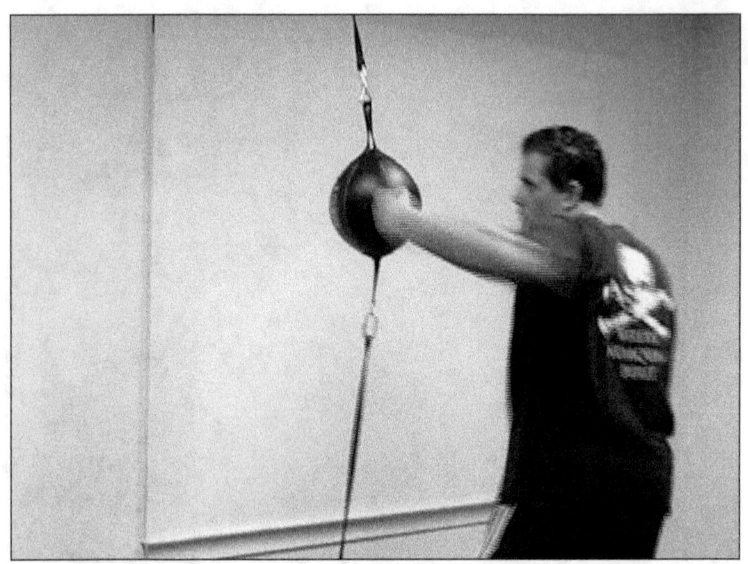

Step 5: Throw another lead hook at the bag.

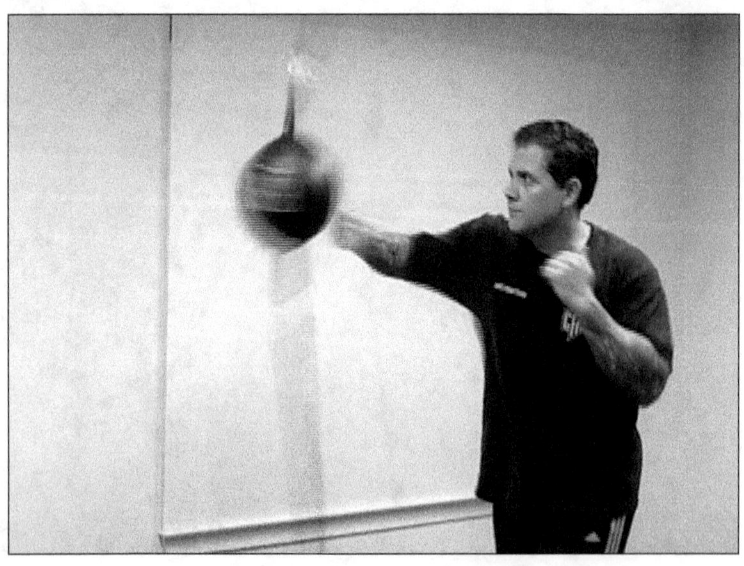

Step 6: Finish with a rear hook.

Combination #8: jab-lead uppercut-rear cross

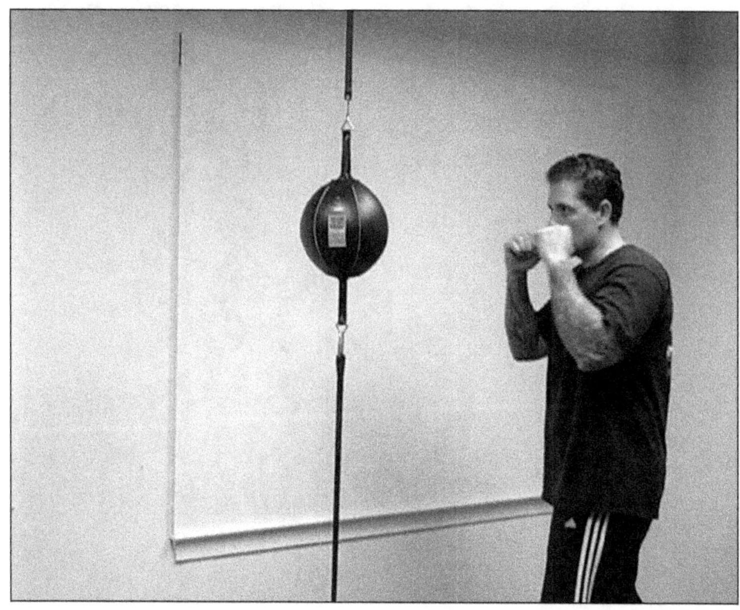

Step 1: Begin from a fighting stance.

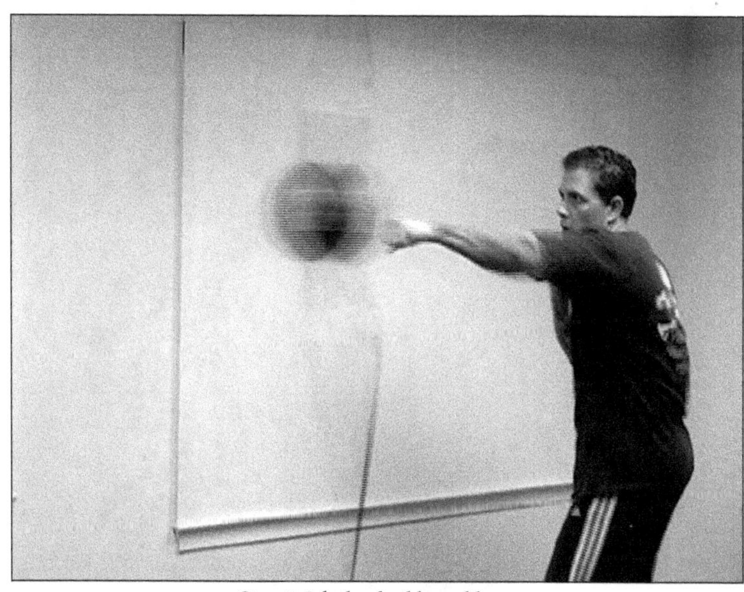

Step 2: Jab the double end bag.

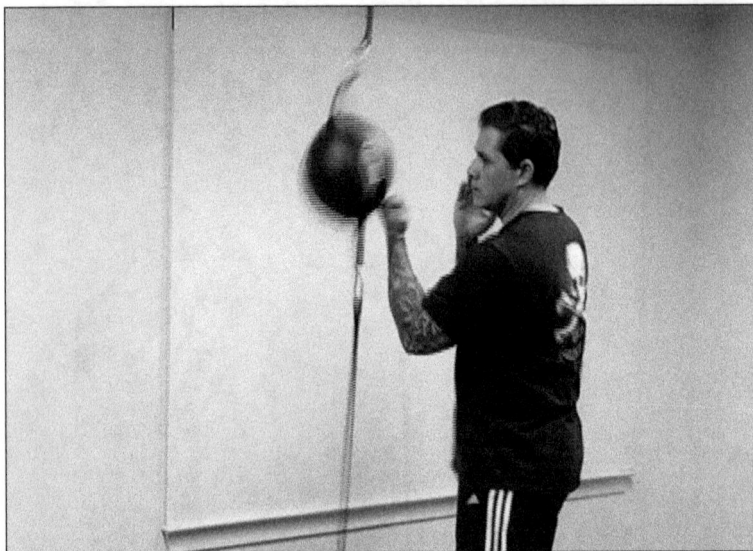

Step 3: With the same arm, throw a lead uppercut.

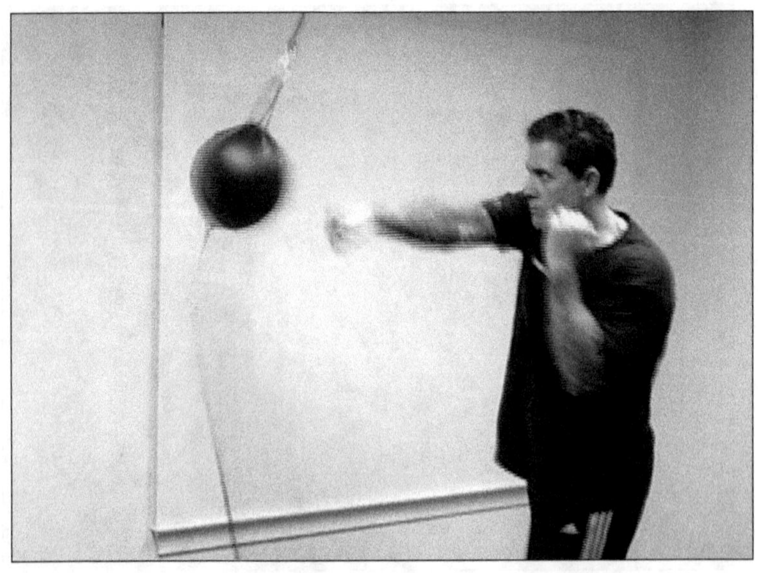

Step 4: Follow up with a rear cross.

Combination #9: jab-rear cross-lead & rear hooks-lead & rear uppercuts

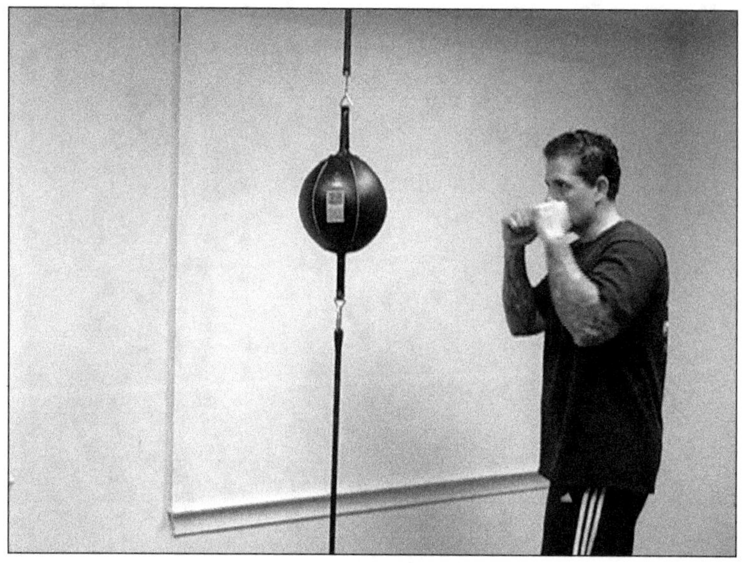

Step 1: Begin from a fighting stance.

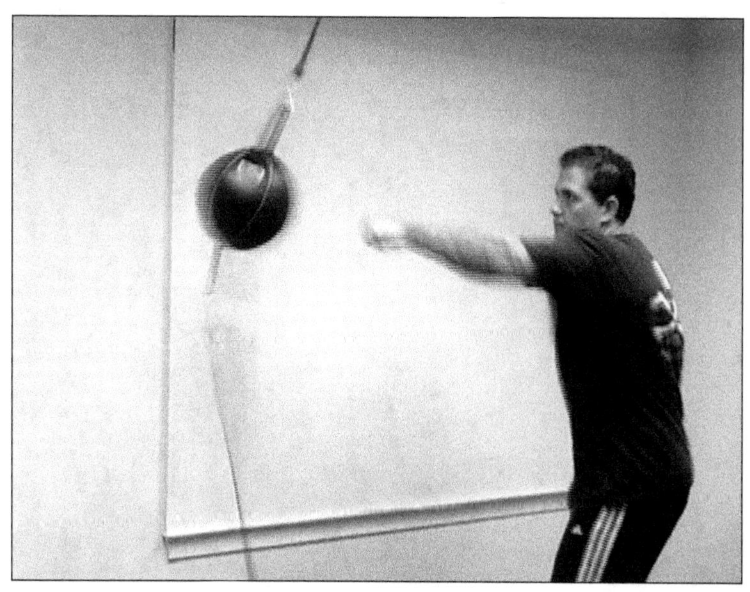

Step 2: Jab at the bag.

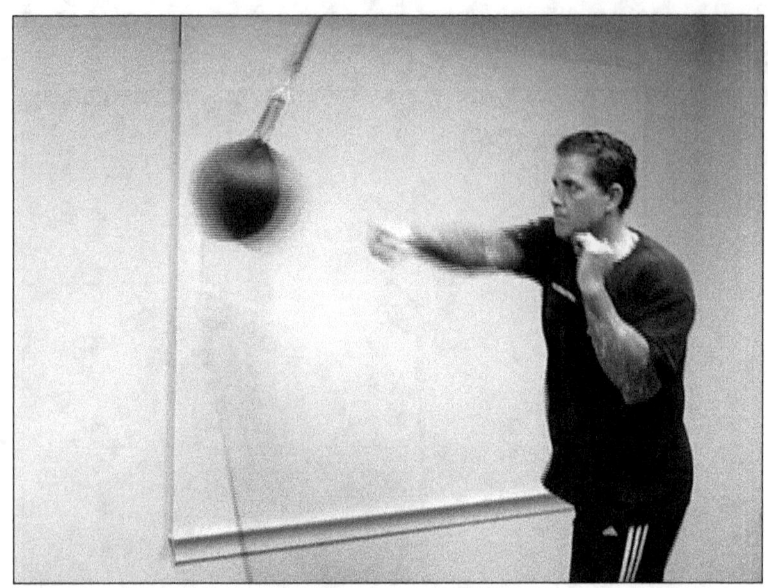

Step 3: Throw a high rear cross.

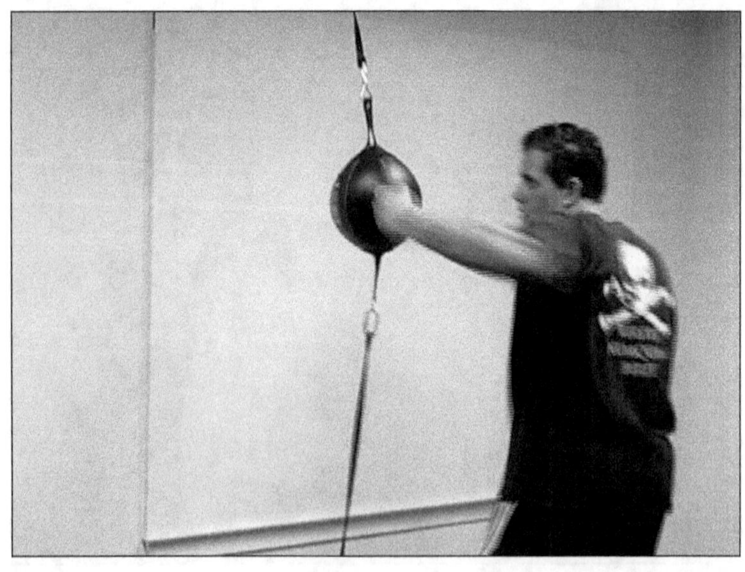

Step 4: Next, a lead hook.

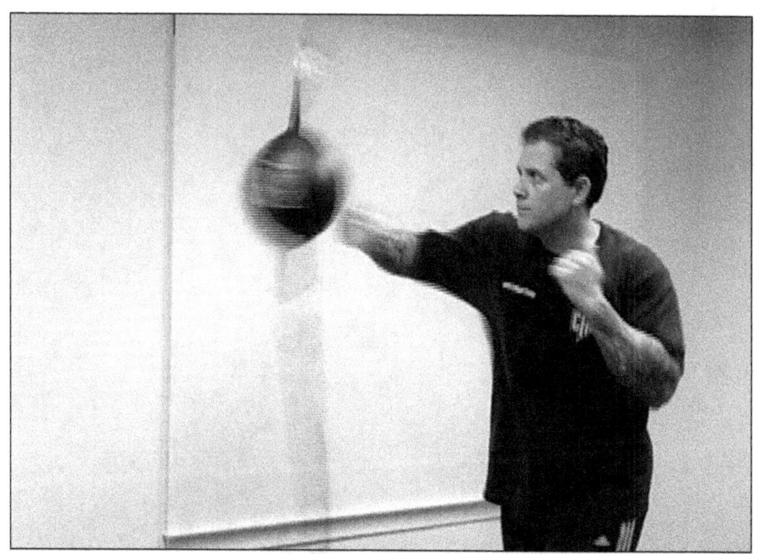

Step 5: Deliver a rear hook.

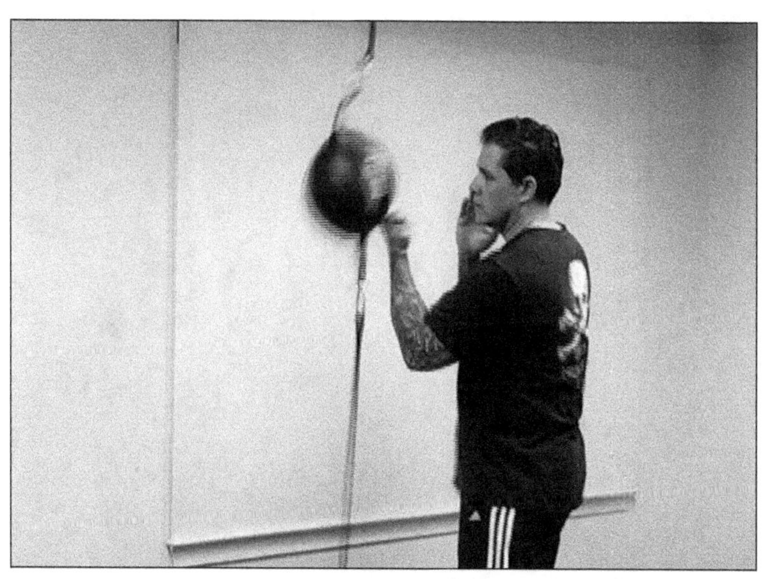

Step 6: A lead uppercut.

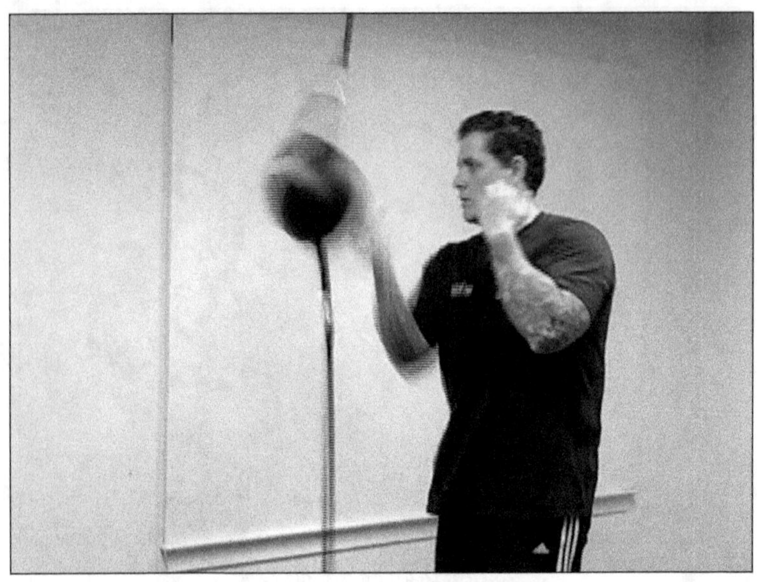

Step 7: Follow with a rear uppercut.

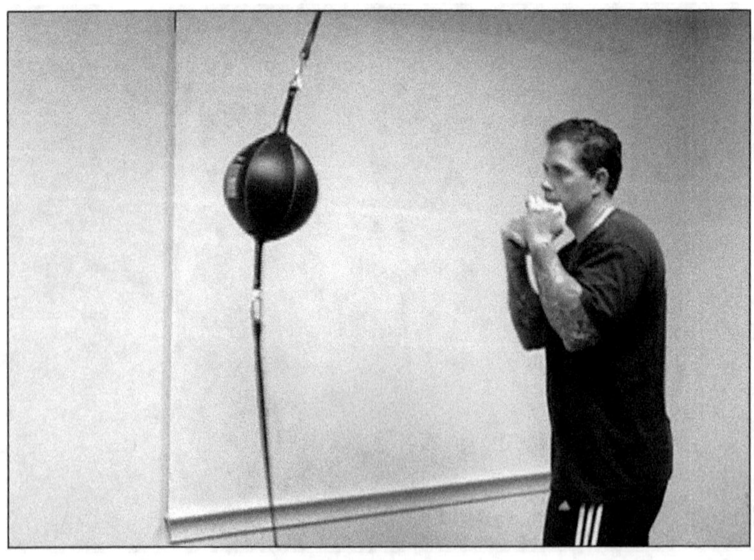

Step 8: Return to your fighting stance.

Workout Routine #2
Ambidextrous Training

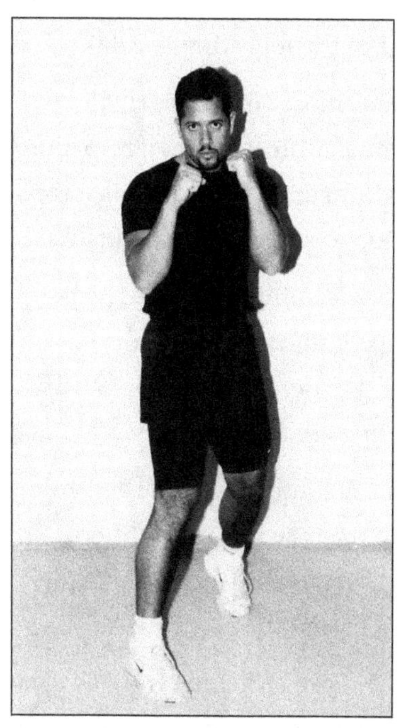
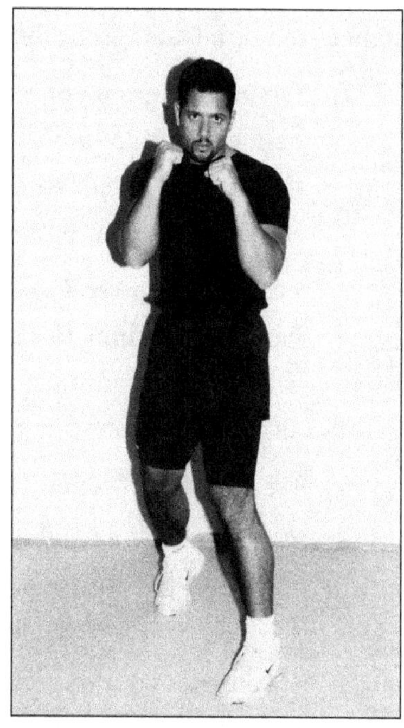

Ambidexterity is the ability to perform with equal facility on both the right and left sides of the body. In simpler terms, it's the capacity to use the right and left hands equally well.

Ambidexterity is a vital attribute for reality-based self-defense training. In fact, it's a regular part of my teaching curriculum. Here are three important reasons why: (1) your strong or dominant hand might be injured in combat, (2) you might be assaulted on the weak side of your body, and (3) your strong hand might be occupied (i.e., holding or carrying an object) during the moment of the assault.

Ambidexterity for Boxing and Mixed Martial Arts

Ambidexterity is also an invaluable skill for combat sports like boxing, kickboxing, and mixed martial arts. In fact, the ability to fight your opponent from both right (southpaw) and left (orthodox) stances can be advantageous for some of the following reasons.

1. **Opens the opponent up** - Since most boxers are right-handed, they are used to fighting against other right-handed fighters. However, switching from an orthodox to a southpaw stance opens your opponent up to several angular attacks.
2. **Lead hand power & accuracy** - Assuming you are right-handed, switching to a southpaw stance places your most accurate and coordinated hand closer to the opponent. This allows you to jab with greater power and accuracy.
3. **Weak hand power enhancer** - A southpaw stance also brings your weaker left hand back to the rear side of your body. This means greater impact power when delivering rear punches (i.e., rear cross, hook, and uppercut).
4. **It confuses your opponent** - Finally, switching from an orthodox to a southpaw stance (in the middle if a fight) will undoubtedly confuse the hell out of your opponent and throw off his timing and footwork. In most cases, it will take a couple rounds for him to get his bearing straight. This creates an enormous window of opportunity that you can exploit to your advantage.

Ambidexterity and Double End Bag Training

There are numerous ways you can incorporate ambidexterity training to your double end bag workouts. Here are just a few.

1. **Switch after every round** - Begin your first round on the double end bag from an orthodox (left lead) stance and

deliver all of your punching combinations from this position. During the next round, switch to a southpaw (right lead) stance and deliver all of your combinations from this posture. Every round, switch between right and left stances for a total of 8 to 10 rounds.

2. **Switch after every combination** - Deliver a specific combination (i.e., jab-rear cross-lead hook-rear hook) from an orthodox stance. Next, switch to a southpaw stance and perform the same bag combination. Switch back to the orthodox stance and perform another combination. Once again, change to a southpaw stance and deliver the same combination on the bag. Go back and forth between stances for the duration of your round. Perform this for a total of 8 to 10 rounds.
3. **Switch after circling** - From an orthodox stance, deliver a series of combinations while rotating 360-degrees around the double end bag. Once your circle is complete, switch to a southpaw stance and execute a series of combinations while circling the opposite direction around the bag. Switch back and forth between right and left stances for a total of 8 to 10 rounds.

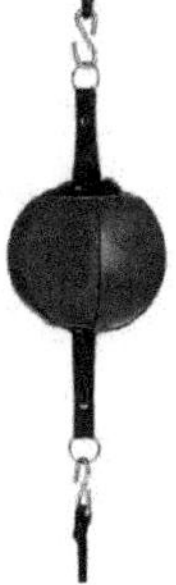

While many boxing purists will argue against switching stances, there are others who disagree. For example, professional boxers like Marvin Hagler, Michael Moorer, Roy Jones Jr., Manny Pacquiao, and Erik Morales are known for switching their stances during a match.

Ambidextrous Training
Switching Your Stance After Every Round

Round	Stance	Round Duration	Rest Period
1	orthodox	3 minutes	1 minute
2	southpaw	3 minutes	1 minute
3	orthodox	3 minutes	1 minute
4	southpaw	3 minutes	1 minute
5	orthodox	3 minutes	1 minute
6	southpaw	3 minutes	1 minute
7	orthodox	3 minutes	1 minute
8	southpaw	3 minutes	1 minute
9	orthodox	3 minutes	1 minute
10	southpaw	3 minutes	1 minute

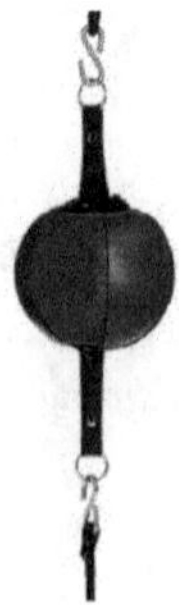

Some boxing coaches and trainers will argue that it's too difficult for a fighter to maintain two stances. However, I categorically disagree! As a matter of fact, I've maintained fighting proficiency with both the right and left stances for over 30 years. The bottom line is, if you want something bad enough, you can make it happen!

Switching After Every Combination

Stance	Combination Sequence
orthodox	Jab (high) - Jab (high)
southpaw	Jab (high) - Jab (high)
orthodox	Jab (high) - Jab (low)
southpaw	Jab (high) - Jab (low)
orthodox	Jab (high) - Jab (high) - Rear Cross (low)
southpaw	Jab (high) - Jab (high) - Rear Cross (low)
orthodox	Jab - Rear Cross - Lead Hook (high)
southpaw	Jab - Rear Cross - Lead Hook (high)
orthodox	Jab - Rear Cross - Lead Hook (low) - Rear Hook (low)
southpaw	Jab - Rear Cross - Lead Hook (low) - Rear Hook (low)
orthodox	Jab - Lead Hook (low) - Rear hook (low)
southpaw	Jab - Lead Hook (low) - Rear hook (low)
orthodox	Jab - Jab - Rear Cross - Lead Hook (high)
southpaw	Jab - Jab - Rear Cross - Lead Hook (high)
orthodox	Rear Cross - Lead Hook - Lead Hook - Rear Hook (all high)
southpaw	Rear Cross - Lead Hook - Lead Hook - Rear Hook (all high)

Note: "low" represents punches delivered to the lower bag when using a double-double end bag or a Mexican style double end bag.

Switching After Circling		
Stance	**Combination Sequence**	**Direction of Movement**
orthodox	Jab (high) - Jab (high)	Circle left
southpaw	Jab (high) - Jab (high)	Circle right
orthodox	Jab (high) - Jab (low)	Circle left
southpaw	Jab (high) - Jab (low)	Circle right
orthodox	Jab (high) - Jab (high) - Rear Cross (low)	Circle left
southpaw	Jab (high) - Jab (high) - Rear Cross (low)	Circle right
orthodox	Jab - Rear Cross - Lead Hook (high)	Circle left
southpaw	Jab - Rear Cross - Lead Hook (high)	Circle right
orthodox	Jab - Rear Cross - Lead Hook (low) - Rear Hook (low)	Circle left
southpaw	Jab - Rear Cross - Lead Hook (low) - Rear Hook (low)	Circle right
orthodox	Jab - Lead Hook (low) - Rear hook (low)	Circle left
southpaw	Jab - Lead Hook (low) - Rear hook (low)	Circle right
orthodox	Jab - Jab - Rear Cross - Lead Hook (high)	Circle left
southpaw	Jab - Jab - Rear Cross - Lead Hook (high)	Circle right
orthodox	Rear Cross - Lead Hook - Lead Hook - Rear Hook (all high)	Circle left
southpaw	Rear Cross - Lead Hook - Lead Hook - Rear Hook (all high)	Circle right

Workout Routine #3
Piston Punching

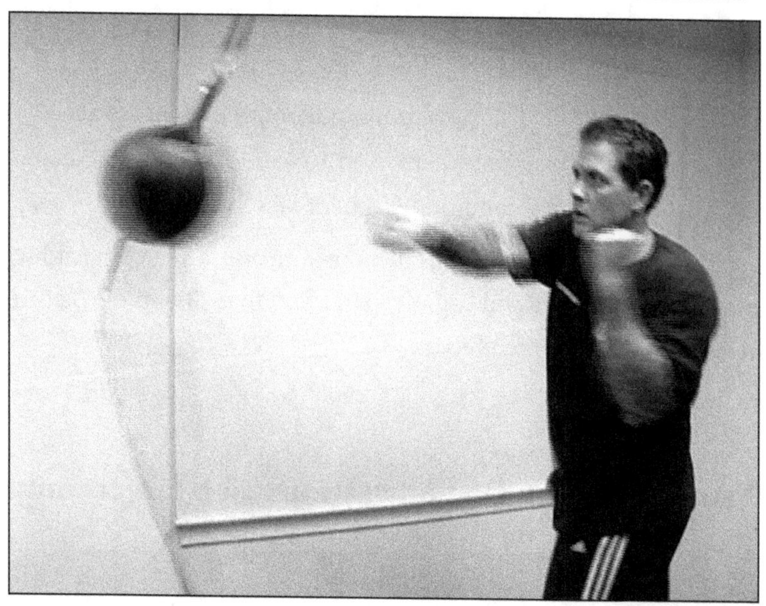

Piston Punching is another challenging double end bag exercise that will push you to your limits. Your objective is to fire off linear punches in a rapid-fire or piston-like fashion at the bag. Piston punching can be directed to high targets (for a standard double end bag) and low targets (for a double-double end bag or Mexican style double end bag).

This exercise is very taxing on the shoulders, so remember to take your time and gradually increase the intensity of this exercise. To perform piston punching, follow these steps:

1. Face the double end bag and assume a fighting stance.
2. Deliver the jab and rear cross combination continuously. Concentrate on delivering full-speed punches.

3. Focus on snapping each punch and *while completely rotating your hips and shoulders.* If the double end bag spins when performing this exercise, it means your punches are not landing at the center. Remember to focus all of your blows to a single center point on the bag.
4. Perform the drill for a minimum of three rounds. Each round can last anywhere from 10 to 60 seconds. If you are exceptionally conditioned, go for 90 seconds.

The following photographs demonstrate piston punching at high targets on the double end bag. Keep in mind that all of these pictures were taken in real-time speed.

Piston Punching Demonstration (high targets only)

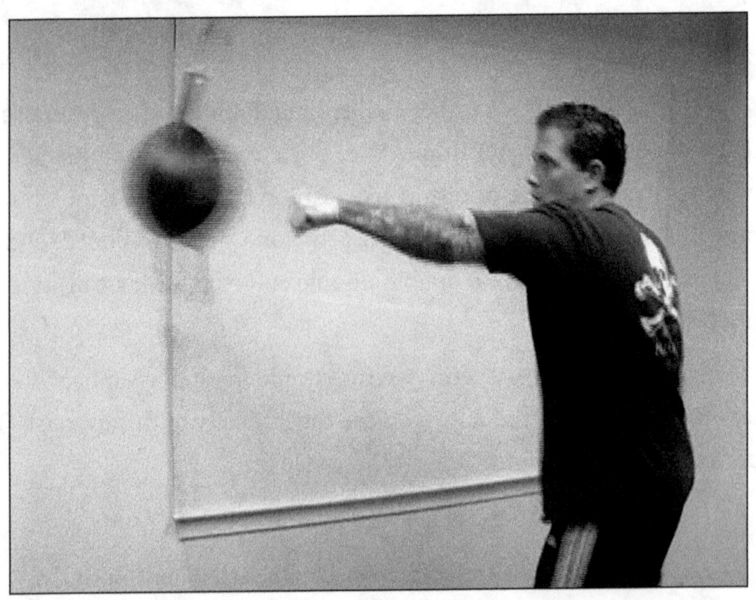

Step 1: The drill begins with a quick jab at the bag.

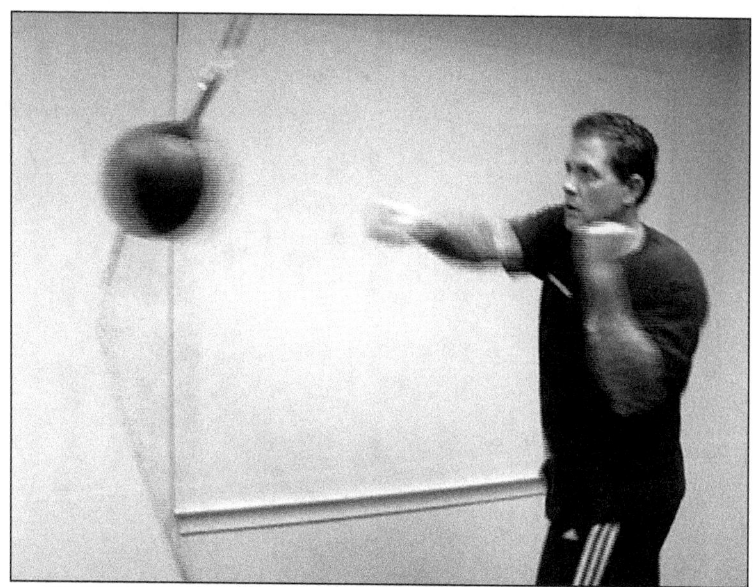

Step 2: Followed by a rear cross.

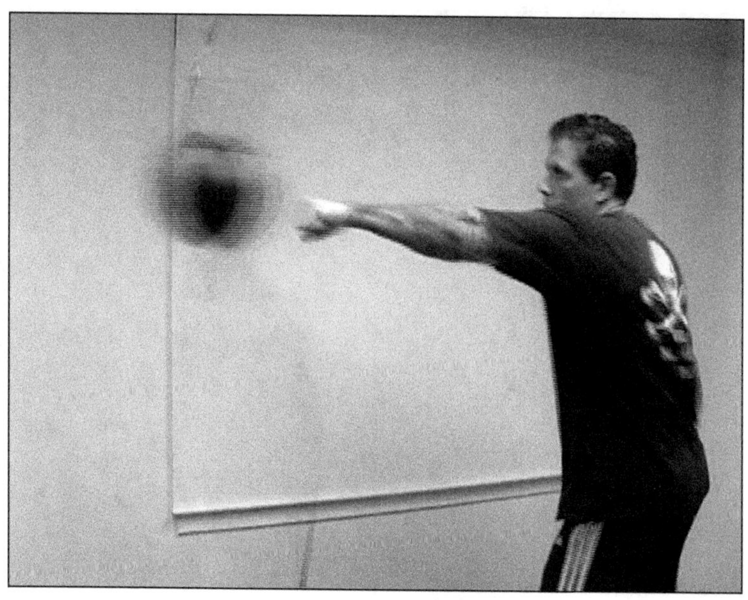

Step 3: Next, another quick jab.

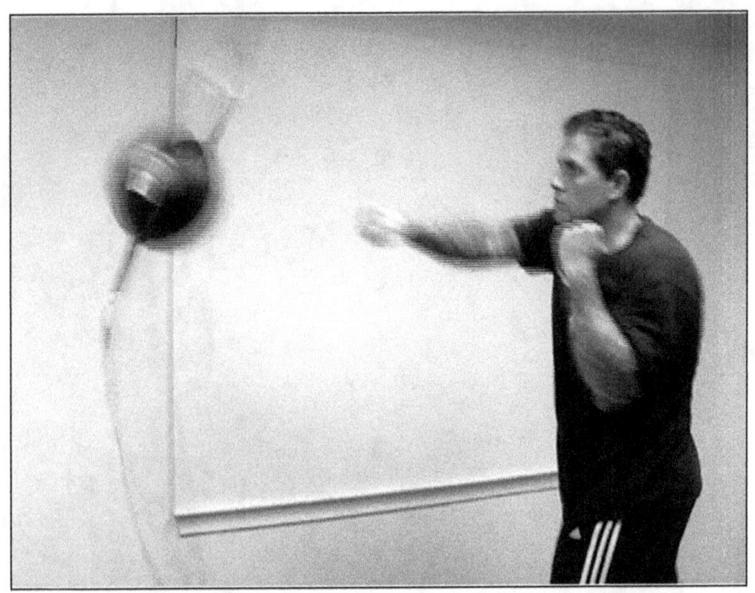

Step 4: The author continues with another rear cross at the bag.

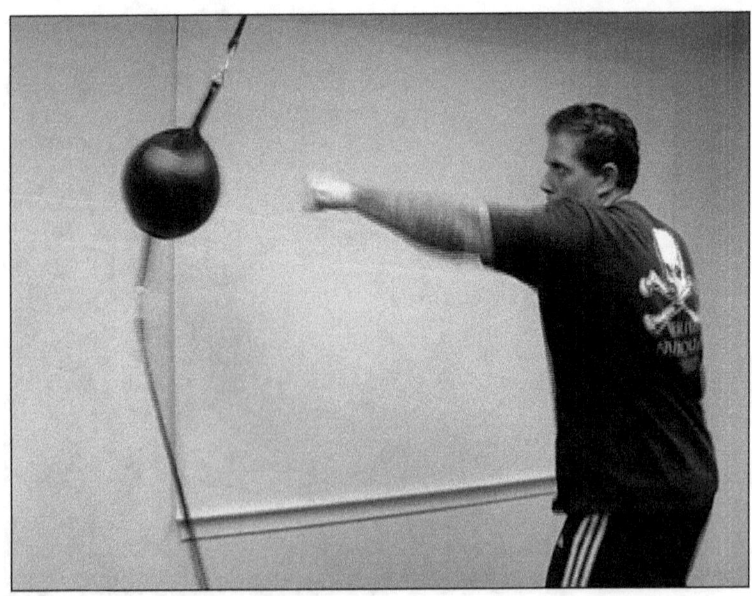

Step 5: He follows up with another jab.

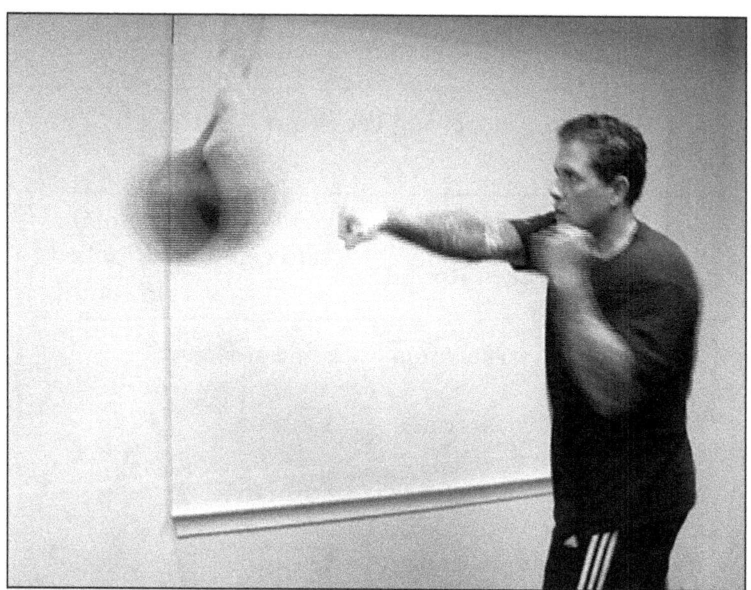

Step 6: Next, another rear cross. Notice how he maintains control of the bag throughout the exercise.

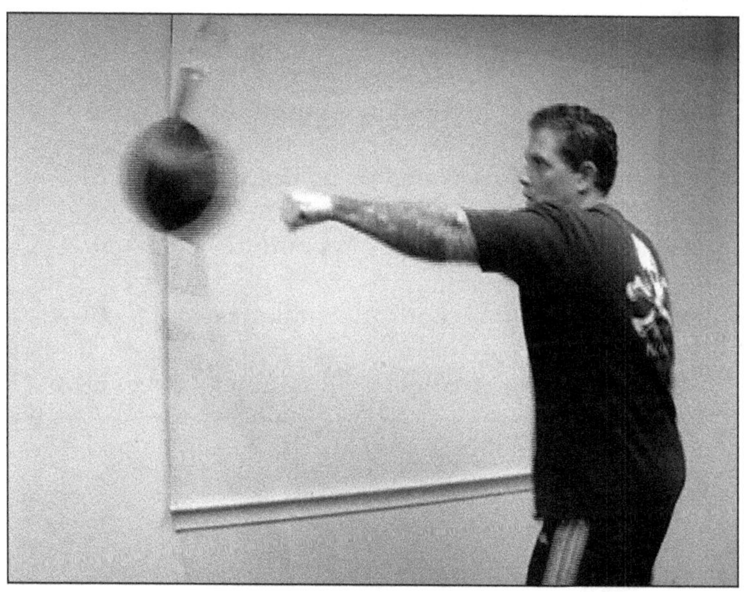

Step 8: Mr. Franco continues his assault for a total of 30 seconds.

Piston Punching Workout Routines

Skill Level	Duration of Each Round	Rest Period	Total Number of rounds
Beginner	10 seconds	2 minutes	3
Beginner	15 seconds	1 minute	3
Beginner	20 seconds	2 minutes	3
Beginner	25 minutes	1 minute	3
Intermediate	30 seconds	2 minutes	5
Intermediate	35 seconds	1 minute	5
Intermediate	40 seconds	2 minutes	5
Intermediate	45 seconds	1 minute	5
Advanced	60 seconds	2 minutes	6
Advanced	70 seconds	1 minute	6
Advanced	80 seconds	2 minutes	6
Advanced	90 seconds	1 minute	6

Workout Routine #4
Cyclone Drill

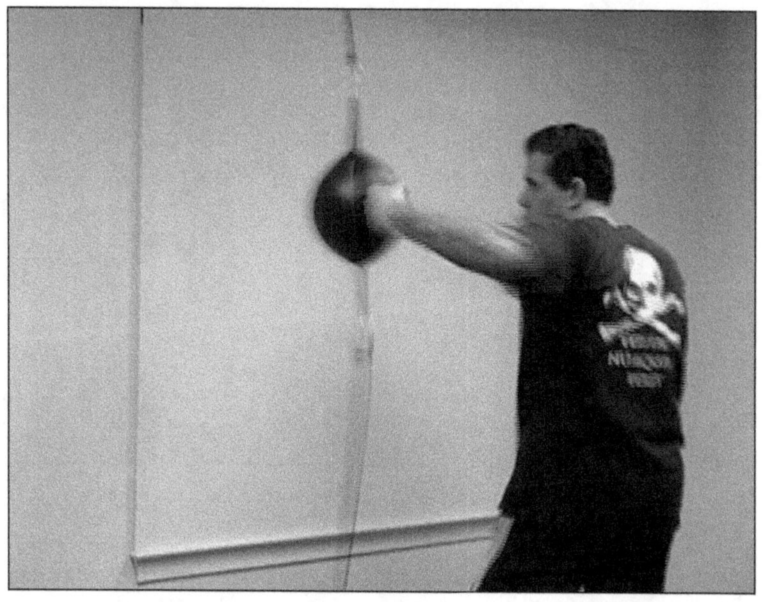

The objective of the exercise is to assault the double end bag with a flurry of hook punches delivered in a back and forth fashion. To perform the Cyclone drill, follow these steps:

1. Face the double end bag and assume a fighting stance.
2. Deliver the lead and rear hook punches in a fluid, back and forth fashion. Timing is critical so try to remain loose and relaxed.
3. Remember to maintain proper punching form throughout the duration of the drill.
4. Perform the exercise for a minimum of three rounds. Each round can last anywhere from 10 to 90 seconds.

Cyclone Drill Demonstration

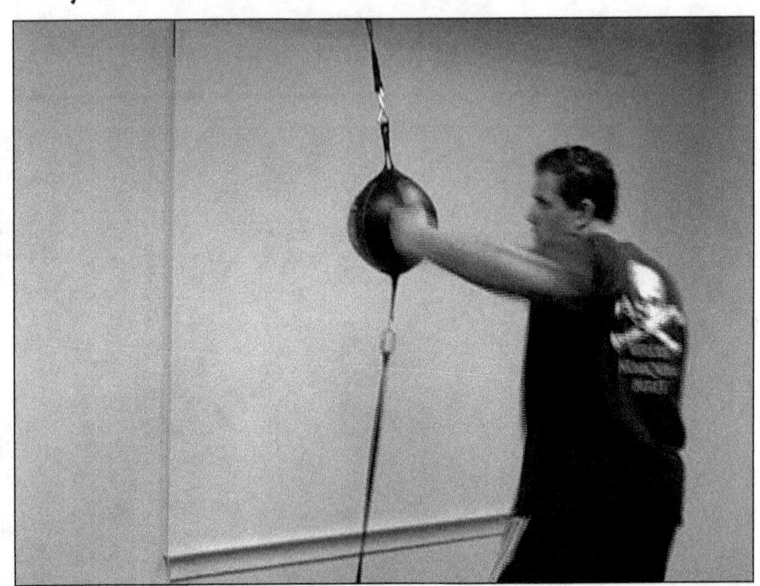

Step 1: The practitioner throws a high lead hook punch at the bag.

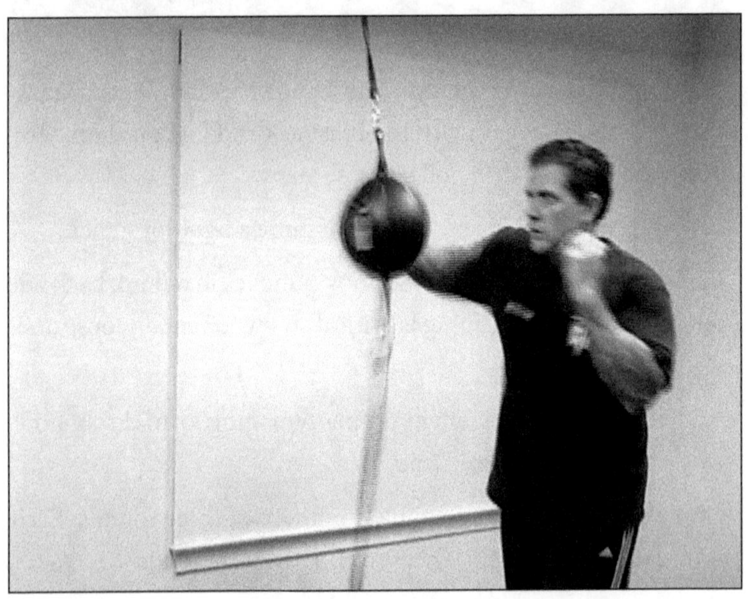

Step 2: Next, a rear hook.

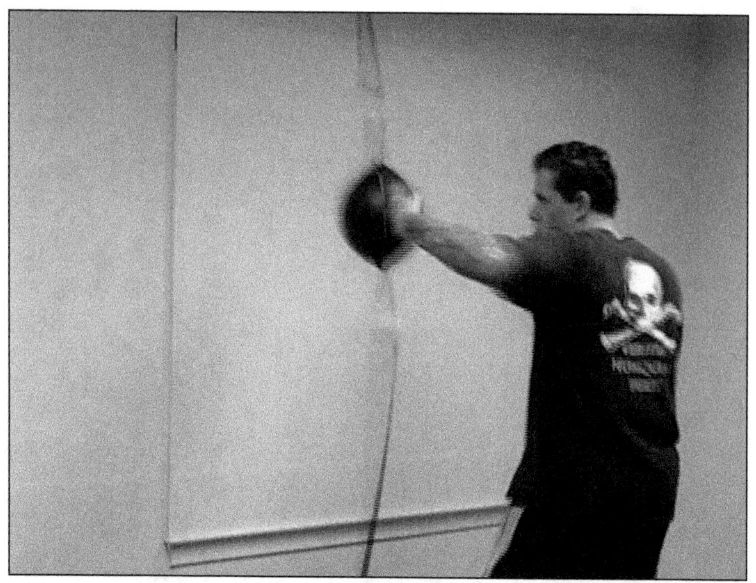

Step 3: Followed by a lead hook.

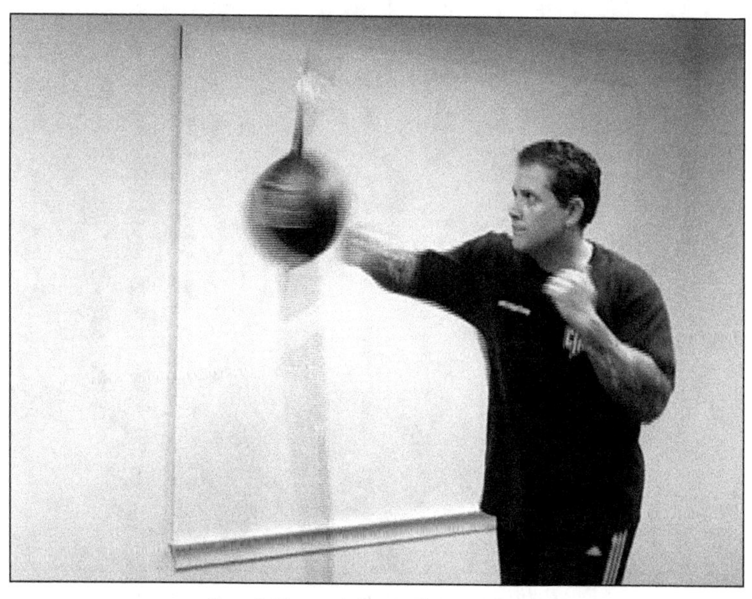

Step 4: He continues with a rear hook.

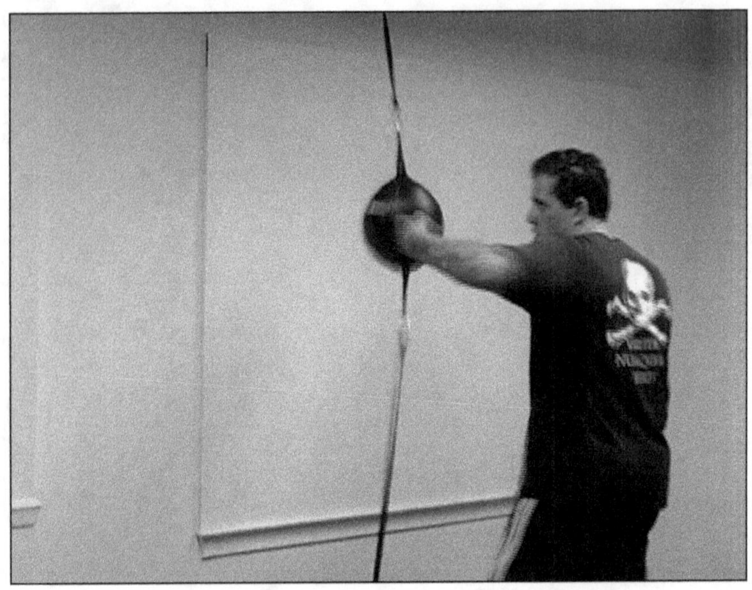

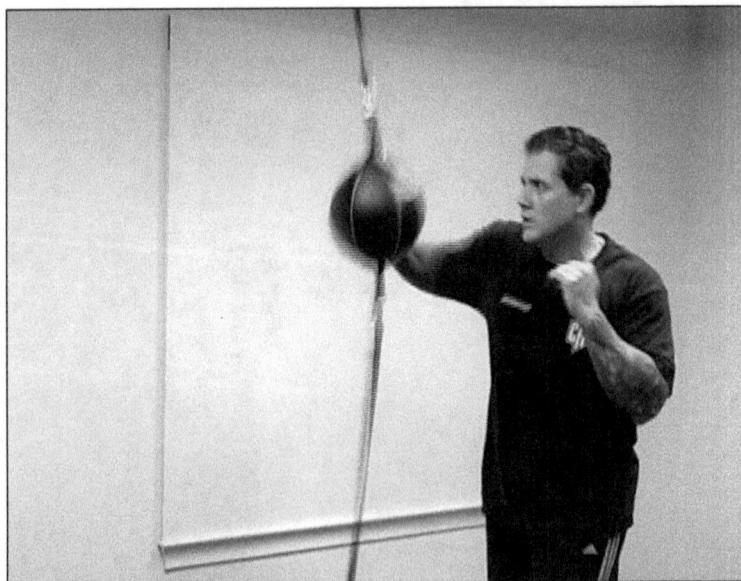

Step 5: Then another high lead hook punch.

Step 6: The practitioner continues his assault for a total of 30 seconds.

Cyclone Drill Workout Routines

Skill Level	Duration of Each Round	Rest Period	Total Number of rounds
Beginner	10 seconds	2 minutes	3
Beginner	15 seconds	1 minute	3
Beginner	20 seconds	2 minutes	3
Beginner	25 minutes	1 minute	3
Intermediate	30 seconds	2 minutes	5
Intermediate	35 seconds	1 minute	5
Intermediate	40 seconds	2 minutes	5
Intermediate	45 seconds	1 minute	5
Advanced	60 seconds	2 minutes	6
Advanced	70 seconds	1 minute	6
Advanced	80 seconds	2 minutes	6
Advanced	90 seconds	1 minute	6

Workout Routine #5
"Hit the Seam" Drill

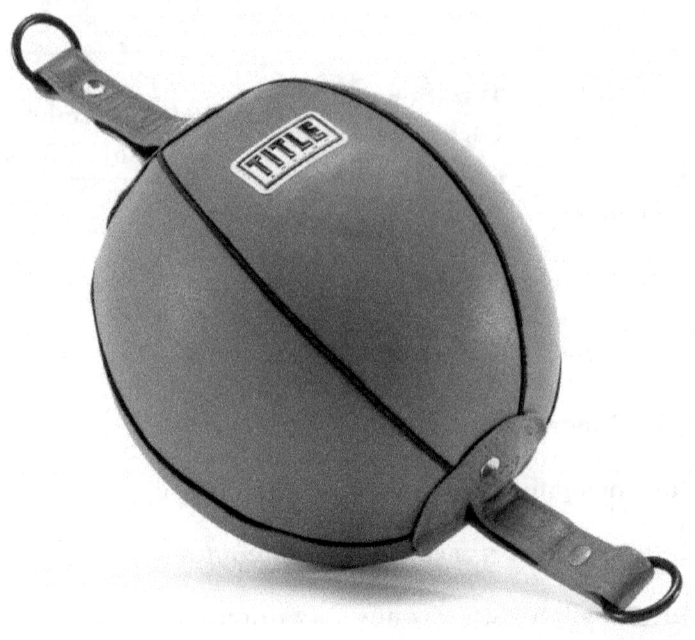

I developed this unusual exercise approximately 25 years ago. My goal was to design a double end bag drill that would help develop *pinpoint* punching accuracy. As you might already know, the double end bag is primarily designed for improving striking accuracy. However, this unique drill takes it to a completely different level.

The objective of "hit the seam" is to deliberately throw punching combinations at the stitching seam that runs vertically down the bag. This is especially challenging because the double end bag swings and spins uncontrollably. So you'll be forced to move continuously with the bag to ensure proper targeting.

"Hit the seam" also develops target recognition along the

opponent's centerline. Essentially, target recognition is the ability to immediately recognize strategic anatomical targets during a fight. Depending on what you are training for (i.e., boxing, mixed martial arts, kickboxing, military combatives, street fighting, etc), the opponent's targets might include his eyes, temple, nose, chin, back of neck, throat, solar plexus, ribs, groin, thighs, knees, and shins.

The Centerline

"Hit the seam" is also ideal for teaching you how to strike the opponent's centerline. The centerline is an imaginary vertical line that divides the opponent's body in half. Located on this line are some of his vital impact targets. This includes the eyes, nose, chin, throat, solar plexus, and groin. Striking these centerline targets in a fight will disrupt your opponent's balance, inhibit his mobility and maximize impact damage. However, combat sports like boxing, mixed martial arts, and kickboxing have rules and regulations that will limit which centerline targets you can strike.

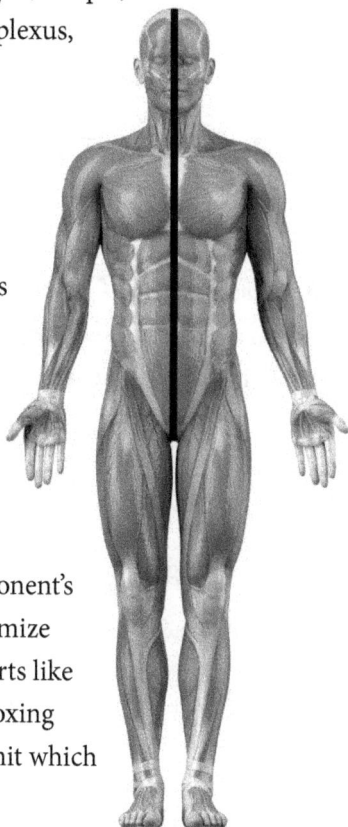

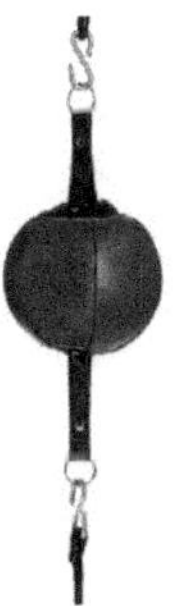

The proper placement of your centerline (in relation to your opponent) is also important and will directly effect your target exposure, balance, mobility, and punching power.

"Hit the Seam" Drill Variations

There are three variations of this drill, and they are listing in order of increased difficulty:

1. **Hit the Seam - straight punches only**
2. **Hit the Seam - circular punches only**
3. **Hit the Seam - all punches**

"Hit the Seam" - Straight Punches Only

This is the easiest of all three variations. It requires you to only throw linear combinations (i.e., jab-jab-rear cross-jab) at the double end bag seam. Also, if you are using a double-double end bag or a Mexican style double end bag you can throw low straight punches at the bag. Here are some punching combinations to get you started.

- Jab (high) - Jab (high)
- Jab (low) - Jab (low)
- Jab (high) - Jab (low)
- Jab (low) - Jab (high)
- Jab (high) - Jab (high) - Rear Cross (high)
- Jab (high) - Jab (high) - Rear Cross (low)
- Jab - Rear Cross (high)
- Jab - Rear Cross (low)
- Jab - Rear Cross (high) - Jab
- Jab - Rear Cross (low) - Jab
- Jab - Rear Cross - Jab - Rear Cross

- Jab - Jab - Rear Cross
- Jab - Rear Cross - Jab

"Hit the Seam" - Circular Punches Only

This drill variation requires an intermediate level of double end bag skill. The goal is to only throw circular punches (hooks, shovel hooks, and uppercuts) at the stitching seam of the double end bag. Again, if you are using a double-double end bag or a Mexican style bag, you can throw circular punches at both high and low targets. Punching combinations can include some of the following:

- Lead Hook (high) - Rear Hook (high)
- Lead Hook (low) - Lead Hook (low)
- Lead Hook (high) - Rear Hook (low)
- Lead Hook (low) -Rear Hook (high)
- Lead Hook (high) - Lead Hook (high) - Rear Hook (high)
- Lead Hook (high) - Lead Hook (high) - Rear Hook (low)
- Lead Hook (high) - Rear Uppercut (low)
- Lead Hook (high) - - Rear Hook (high) - Rear Uppercut (low)
- Rear Uppercut (low) - Lead Uppercut (low)
- Rear Uppercut (low) - Lead Uppercut (low) - Lead Hook (high) - Rear Hook (high)
- Rear Uppercut (high) - Lead Uppercut (high) - Lead Hook (low) - Rear Hook (low)

"Hit the Seam" - All Punches

This is by far the most challenging of the three variations. It requires you to throw your entire punching arsenal at the seam line. This includes the jab, rear cross, hook, shovel hook, and uppercut. Once again, your punches can be delivered to both high and low double end bag targets. Some striking combinations can include:

- Jab - Jab- Rear Uppercut (all high)
- Jab - Lead Uppercut - Rear Cross (all high)
- Jab - Lead Uppercut - Rear Cross (low-high-low)
- Jab - Rear Uppercut - Lead Uppercut (all high)
- Jab - Rear Uppercut - Lead Uppercut - Rear Cross - Lead Hook (all high)
- Jab - Rear Cross - Lead Hook - Rear Uppercut (all high)
- Jab - Rear Cross - Lead Hook - Rear Cross (all high)
- Jab - rear cross - Lead Hook - Rear Cross - Lead Hook - Lead Hook (5x high -1 low)
- Rear Cross - Jab - Rear Hook (all high)
- Rear Cross - Jab - Rear Hook -Lead Uppercut - Lead Hook (high-high-low-high-high)
- Rear Cross - Lead Hook - Rear Cross - Lead Hook - Rear Uppercut (high-high-high-low-high)
- Rear Hook - Lead Hook - Rear Hook - Lead Uppercut (all high)

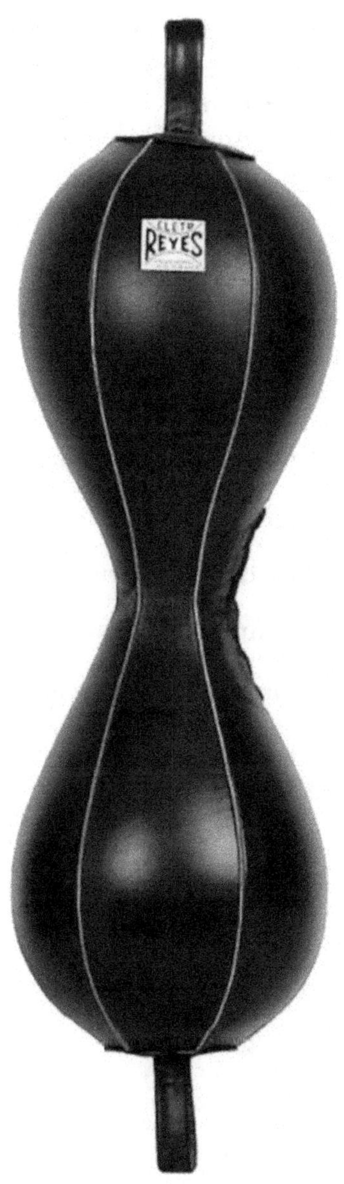

Since the seam runs vertically down the Mexican style double end bag, you can throw both high and low punching combinations.

"Hit the Seam" Workout Routines

Skill Level	Duration of Each Round	Rest Period	Total Number of rounds
Beginner	1 minute	2 minutes	3
Beginner	1 minute	1 minute	3
Beginner	2 minutes	2 minutes	3
Beginner	2 minutes	1 minute	3
Intermediate	3 minutes	2 minutes	5
Intermediate	3 minutes	1 minute	5
Intermediate	3 minutes	2 minutes	6
Intermediate	3 minutes	1 minute	6
Advanced	4 minutes	2 minutes	8
Advanced	4 minutes	1 minute	8
Advanced	5 minutes	2 minutes	10
Advanced	5 minutes	1 minute	10

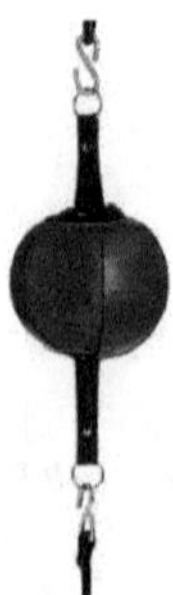

If you want to really push yourself, you can combine different routines into a single workout. For example, try combining ambidextrous training with "hit the seam" drill.

Workout Routine #6
X-Training

X-Training is also another methodology that develops *pinpoint* target accuracy. Compared the previous drill, X-Training is less restrictive. The objective of the exercise is to throw punching combinations at Xs that are on the double end bag.

Preparing the Bag

The best way to prepare your double end bag for X-Training is first to cut several small pieces of white electrical tape into two-inch strips. Next, cross two pieces of tape and form an X and press it firmly into the bag. Space the Xs approximately four to six inches apart from each other and distribute them around the bag.

X-Training Variations

There are three variations of X-Training, and they are listing in order of increased difficulty:

1. **X-Training - straight punches only**
2. **X-Training - circular punches only**
3. **X-Training - all punches**

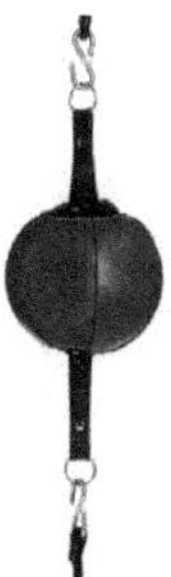

X-Training works equally well with the standard double end bag and the double-double end bag. It's just a matter of personal preference.

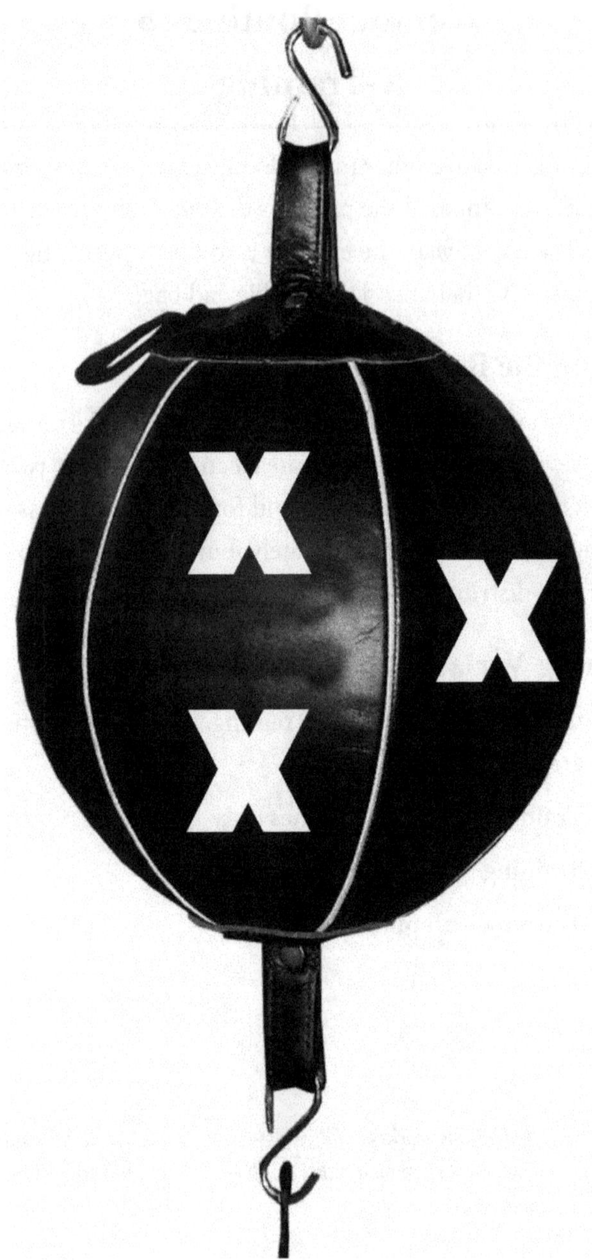

Pictured here, a double end bag prepped for X-Training.

X-Training - Straight Punches Only

This is the easiest of all three variations. It requires you to only throw linear combinations (i.e., jab-jab-rear cross-jab) at the Xs. Again, if you are using a double-double end bag or a Mexican style double end bag you can throw low punches at the bag. Here are some punching combinations to get you started.

- Jab (high) - Jab (high)
- Jab (low) - Jab (low)
- Jab (high) - Jab (low)
- Jab (low) - Jab (high)
- Jab (high) - Jab (high) - Rear Cross (high)
- Jab (high) - Jab (high) - Rear Cross (low)
- Jab - Rear Cross (high)
- Jab - Rear Cross (low)
- Jab - Rear Cross (high) - Jab
- Jab - Rear Cross (low) - Jab
- Jab - Rear Cross - Jab - Rear Cross
- Jab - Jab - Rear Cross
- Jab - Rear Cross - Jab

X-Training - Circular Punches Only

This drill variation requires an intermediate level of double end bag skill. The goal is to only throw circular punches (hooks, shovel hooks, and uppercuts) at the white targets. Punching combinations can include some of the following:

- Lead Hook (high) - Rear Hook (high)
- Lead Hook (low) - Lead Hook (low)
- Lead Hook (high) - Rear Hook (low)
- Lead Hook (low) -Rear Hook (high)
- Lead Hook (high) - Lead Hook (high) - Rear Hook (high)
- Lead Hook (high) - Lead Hook (high) - Rear Hook (low)
- Lead Hook (high) - Rear Uppercut (low)
- Lead Hook (high) - - Rear Hook (high) - Rear Uppercut (low)
- Rear Uppercut (low) - Lead Uppercut (low)
- Rear Uppercut (low) - Lead Uppercut (low) - Lead Hook (high) - Rear Hook (high)
- Rear Uppercut (high) - Lead Uppercut (high) - Lead Hook (low) - Rear Hook (low)

X-Training - All Punches

This is the most challenging of the three variations. It requires you to throw your entire punching arsenal at the Xs. This includes the jab, rear cross, hook, shovel hook, and uppercut. Once again, your punches can be delivered to both high and low double end bag targets. Some striking combinations can include:

- Jab - Jab- Rear Uppercut (all high)
- Jab - Lead Uppercut - Rear Cross (all high)
- Jab - Lead Uppercut - Rear Cross (low-high-low)

- Jab - Rear Uppercut - Lead Uppercut (all high)
- Jab - Rear Uppercut - Lead Uppercut - Rear Cross - Lead Hook (all high)
- Jab - Rear Cross - Lead Hook - Rear Uppercut (all high)
- Jab - Rear Cross - Lead Hook - Rear Cross (all high)
- Jab - rear cross - Lead Hook - Rear Cross - Lead Hook - Lead Hook (5x high -1 low)
- Rear Cross - Jab - Rear Hook (all high)
- Rear Cross - Jab - Rear Hook -Lead Uppercut - Lead Hook (high-high-low-high-high)
- Rear Cross - Lead Hook - Rear Cross - Lead Hook - Rear Uppercut (high-high-high-low-high)
- Rear Hook - Lead Hook - Rear Hook - Lead Uppercut (all high)

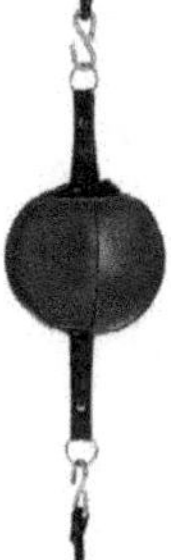

If you are training for a competitive match, always workout on the bag with a mouthpiece in your mouth. Remember, train the way you will fight and fight the way you train!

X-Training
Workout Routines

Skill Level	Duration of Each Round	Rest Period	Total Number of rounds
Beginner	1 minute	2 minutes	3
Beginner	1 minute	1 minute	3
Beginner	2 minutes	2 minutes	3
Beginner	2 minutes	1 minute	3
Intermediate	3 minutes	2 minutes	5
Intermediate	3 minutes	1 minute	5
Intermediate	3 minutes	2 minutes	6
Intermediate	3 minutes	1 minute	6
Advanced	4 minutes	2 minutes	8
Advanced	4 minutes	1 minute	8
Advanced	5 minutes	2 minutes	10
Advanced	5 minutes	1 minute	10

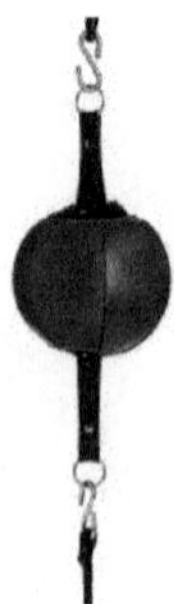

Learn to relax and avoid tensing your muscles when throwing combinations. Muscular tension will throw off your timing, retard the speed of your punches, and wear you out during a round.

Workout Routine #7
Technique Isolation Training

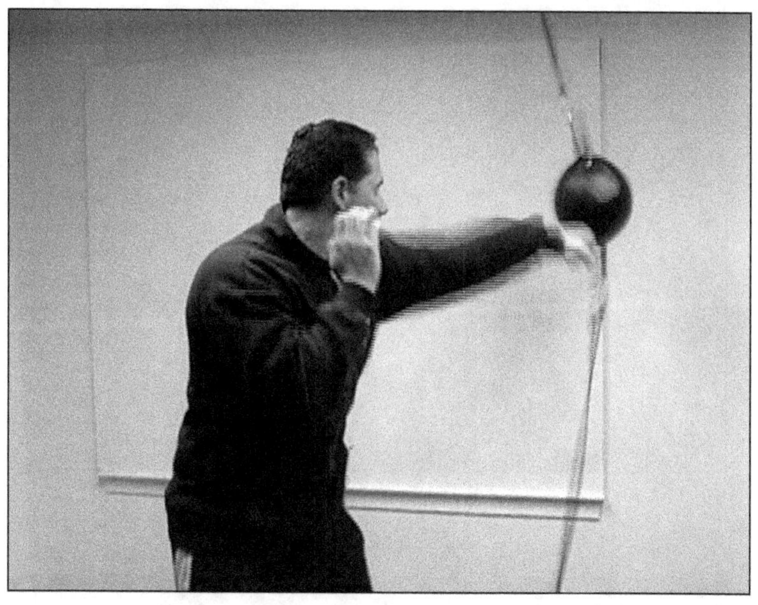

Technique Isolation training is a variation of my proficiency training methodology. The purpose of this exercise is to focus exclusively on one punch (i.e., jab, rear cross, lead hook, etc.) for your entire workout. For example, if you wanted to sharpen and develop your jab, you would isolate and practice it exclusively on the double end bag for a specified number of rounds.

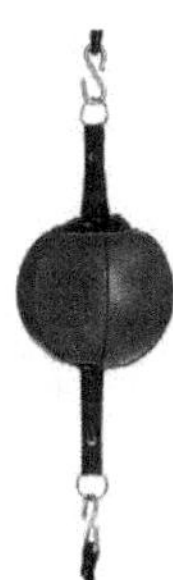

Don't forget to be defensively alert when performing this drill. Arbitrarily slip your head from side to side and always keep your other hand up by your face.

Isolation Training (Jab) Demonstration

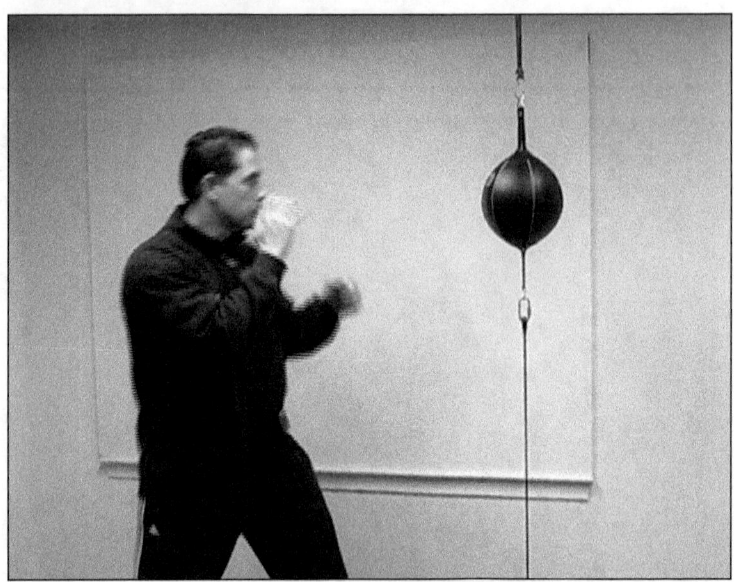

Step 1: The practitioner assumes a stance.

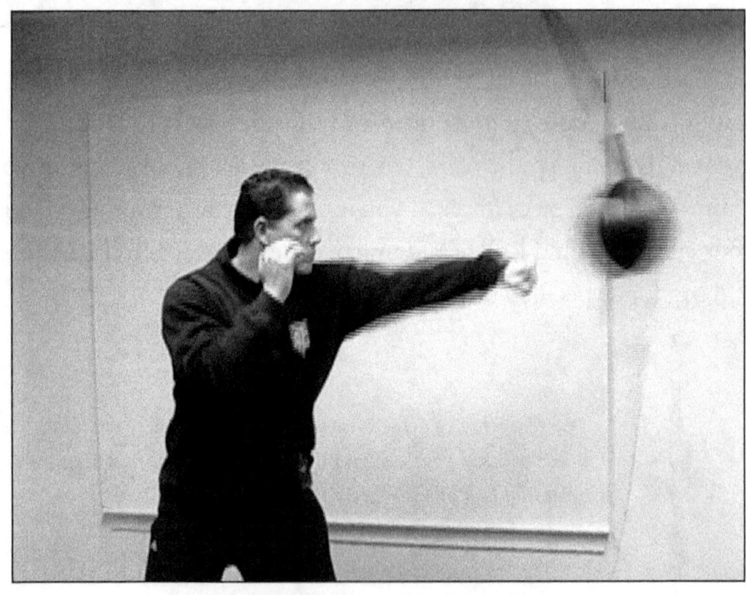

Step 2: He delivers a high left jab.

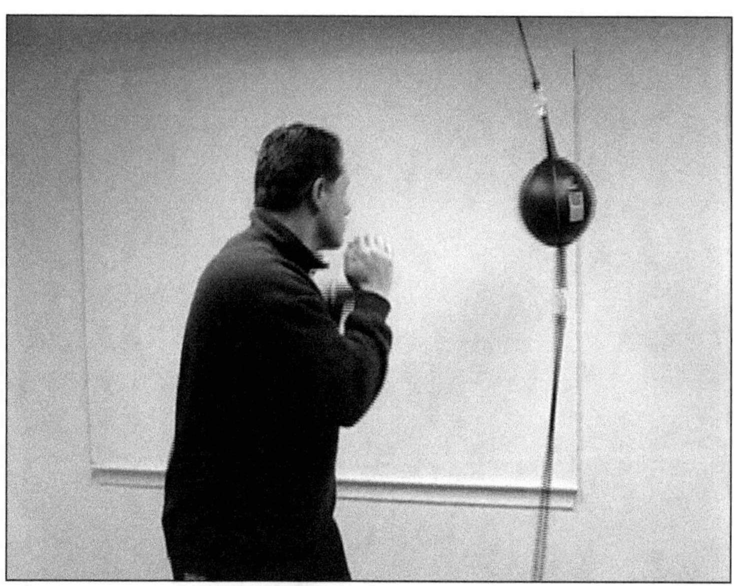

Step 3: He begins circling the bag in a counter clockwise direction.

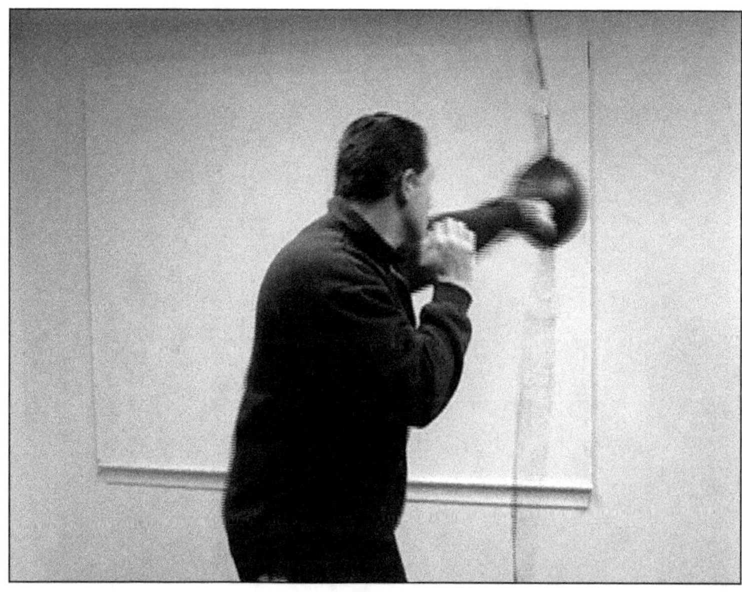

Step 4: He throws another quick jab.

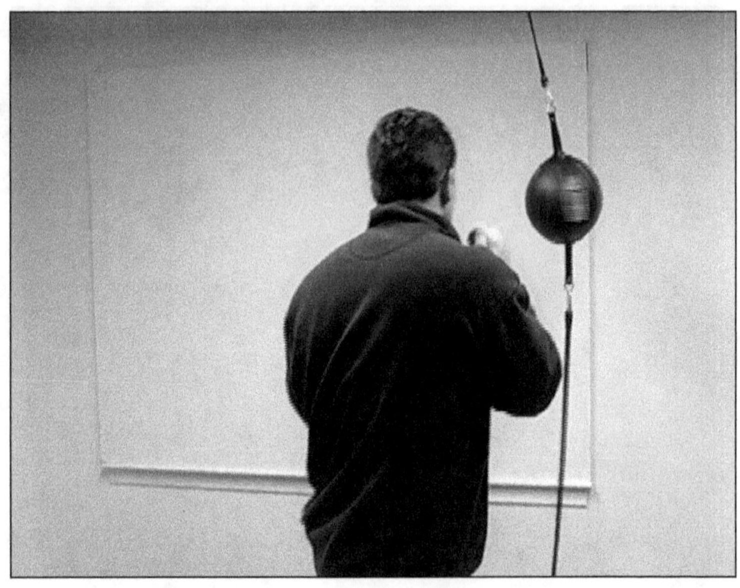

Step 5: Franco continues to move around the double end bag.

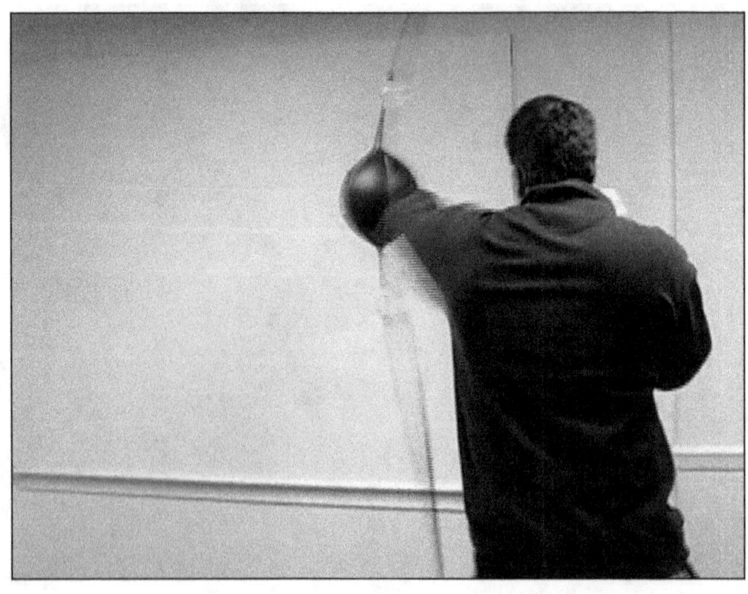

Step 6: Next, another jab.

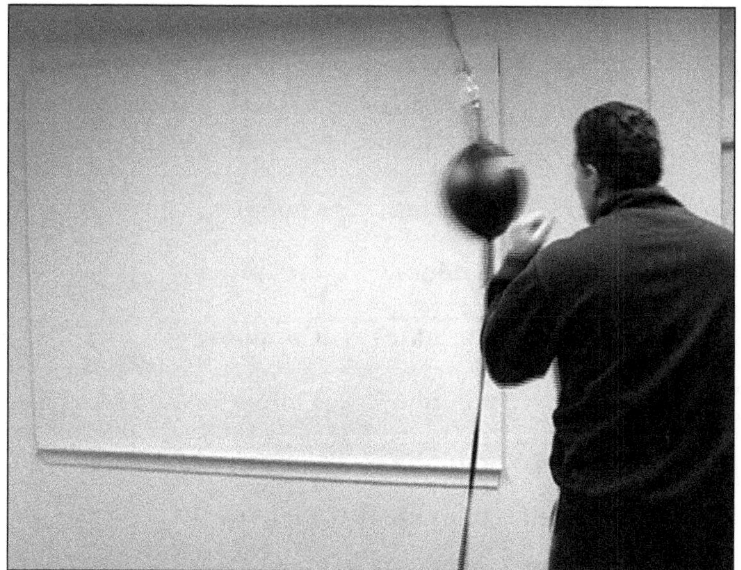

Step 7: The practitioner continues jabbing and moving around the at the bag for a duration of 3 minutes.

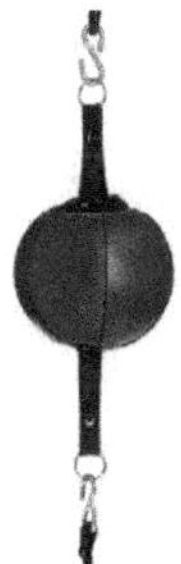

Technique isolation training might seem boring to some people, but it's a sure-fire method of sharpening a particular punching technique.

Technique Isolation Workout Routines

Skill Level	Duration of Each Round	Rest Period	Total Number of rounds
Beginner	1 minute	2 minutes	3
Beginner	1 minute	1 minute	3
Beginner	2 minutes	2 minutes	3
Beginner	2 minutes	1 minute	3
Intermediate	3 minutes	2 minutes	5
Intermediate	3 minutes	1 minute	5
Intermediate	3 minutes	2 minutes	6
Intermediate	3 minutes	1 minute	6
Advanced	4 minutes	2 minutes	8
Advanced	4 minutes	1 minute	8
Advanced	5 minutes	2 minutes	10
Advanced	5 minutes	1 minute	10

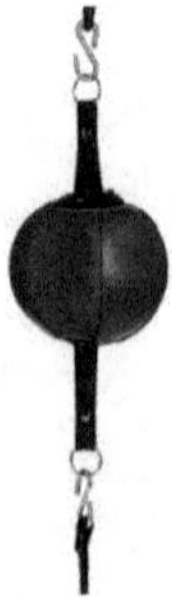

In order to maximize the full benefit of technique isolation training, it's important to stick to only one punch for your entire workout. For example, if you're a beginner who wants to perfect your jab, you would practice it exclusively for a total of 3 rounds.

Workout Routine #8
Defensive Bag Training

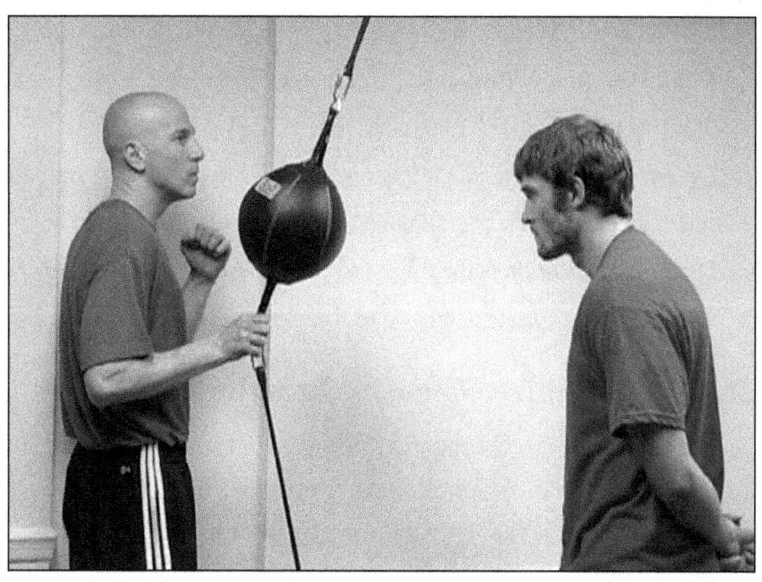

Double end bag training isn't just about offense. In fact, there are several drills designed to sharpen your defensive skills and improve your defensive reaction time.

A good defensive structure requires mastery of the following four tools: blocks, parries, slipping, and footwork. I can say without reservation that all of these defensive techniques work effectively against boxers, street brawlers, and martial artists of all styles and backgrounds. However, before I can discuss the specific defensive tools, it's important to talk about defensive reaction time when fighting.

What is Defensive Reaction Time?

Defensive reaction time is defined as the elapsed time between the opponent's attack (e.g., jab, hook, rear cross) and your defensive response to that attack (e.g., block, parry, evasion movement). Your defensive reaction time is the result of three fluid stages (defensive recognition, defensive selection, and defensive execution).

1. ***Defensive recognition*** is the first stage where you recognize and identify that an attack has occurred.
2. ***Defensive selection*** is the second stage where you immediately select the appropriate defensive tool, technique, or response.
3. ***Defensive execution*** is the third and final phase where your body performs the appropriate defensive tool, technique, or response.

How To Minimize Defensive Reaction Time

When it comes to fighting (including both sport and street), your objective is to minimize your defensive reaction time as much as possible. Luckily, there are several ways to accomplish this.

First, try to be able to read advance information about the opponent's attack. This is referred to as *telegraphic cognizance*. For example, when your opponent chambers his arm back prior to delivering a punch.

Second, limit your number of defensive responses to a particular type of attack. For example, if your opponent attacks with a jab to your head, you should have only *one specific* defensive response programmed. In this instance, you would parry or deflect the threatening blow.

Third, all of your defensive responses should be natural and performed in a simple fashion. Again, in the case of the jab, not only would you execute a horizontal parry, but you would also situate it on the same side of the opponent's attack (this is called mirror-image parrying).

Fourth, practice, practice, practice! Your defensive responses must be practiced over and over again until they become second nature. Sparring, shadowboxing, focus mitt drills, heavy bag and double end bag training will help you develop these important skills.

Before we get into the defensive double end bag exercise, let's review all of the different defensive techniques you would use in a fight.

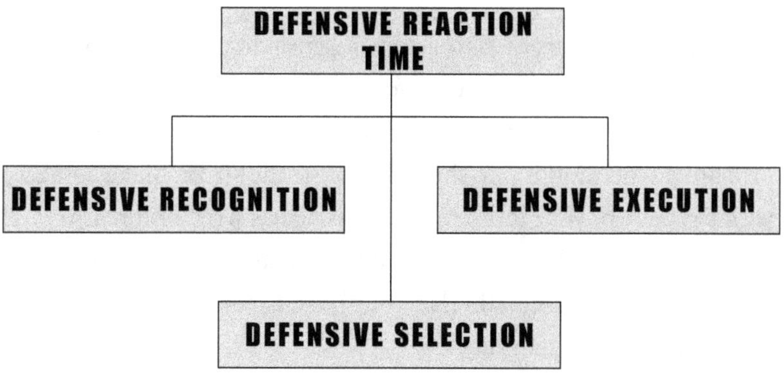

Defensive reaction time is the result of three fluid stages: defensive recognition, defensive selection, and defensive execution.

Arm Blocks

Blocks are defensive techniques designed to intercept your assailant's circular attacks. Blocks are executed by placing a non vital body part between the opponent's strike and your body target. There are three primary blocks with which you need to be proficient. They include high blocks, mid-blocks, and elbow blocks.

High Block

The high block is primarily used for street self-defense and it's designed to protect you against overhead blows. To execute the lead high block, simply raise your lead arm up and extend your forearm out and above your head. Be careful not to position your arm where your head is exposed. Make certain that your hand is open and not clenched. This will increase the surface area of your block and provide a quick counterattack. The mechanics for the lead high block are the same as for the rear high block. Raise your rear arm up and extend your forearm out and above your head.

Mid-Block

The mid-block is used to defend against circular blows to your head or upper torso. To perform the block, raise either your right or left arm at approximately 90 degrees while simultaneously pronating (rotating) it into the direction of the strike. Make contact with the belly of your forearm at the assailant's wrist or forearm. This movement will provide maximum structural integrity for the blocking tool. Make certain that your hand is held open to increase the surface area of your block.

Elbow Block

The elbow block is frequently used in boxing, kickboxing, and mixed martial arts. It's designed to stop circular blows to your midsection, such as uppercuts, shovel hooks, and even hook kicks. To execute the elbow block, drop your elbow and simultaneously twist your body toward your centerline. Be certain to keep your elbow perpendicular to the floor and keep your hands relaxed and close to

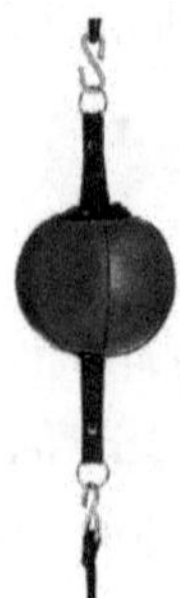

Never forget that offense is only half the game. Defensive skills are just as important and they must be practiced frequently to ensure that you will survive both in the streets and the ring.

your chest. The elbow block can be used on both the right and left sides.

Hand Parries

The parry is a quick, forceful slap that picks-off and redirects your assailant's linear strike (i.e., jab, and rear cross). There are two general types of parries, horizontal and vertical, and both can be executed with the right and left hands.

Horizontal Parry

To properly execute a horizontal parry from a fighting stance, move your lead hand horizontally across your body (centerline) to deflect and redirect the assailant's punch. Immediately return to your

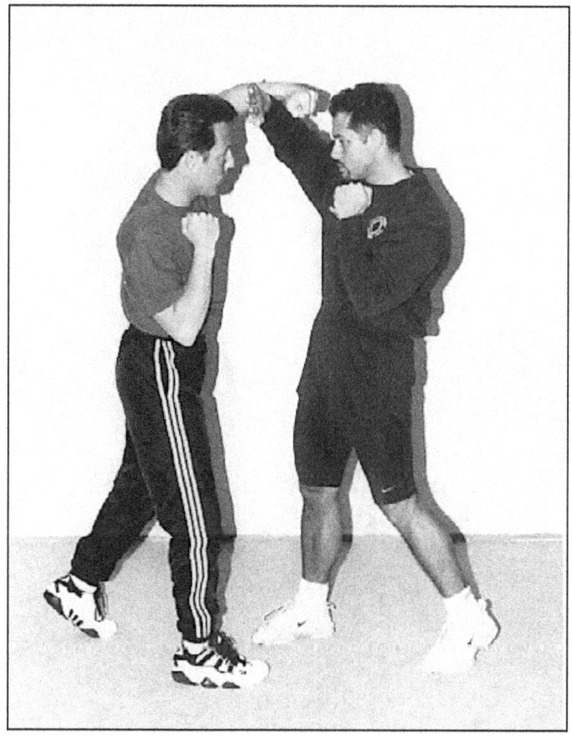

The high block.

guard position. Be certain to make contact with the palm of your hand. With sufficient training, you can effectively incorporate the horizontal parry into slipping maneuvers.

Vertical Parry

To execute a vertical parry, from a fighting stance, move your hand vertically down your body (centerline) to deflect and redirect the assailant's blow. Once again, don't forget to counterattack your assailant. **CAUTION:** *Do not parry with your fingers. The fingers provide no structural integrity, and they can be jammed or broken easily.*

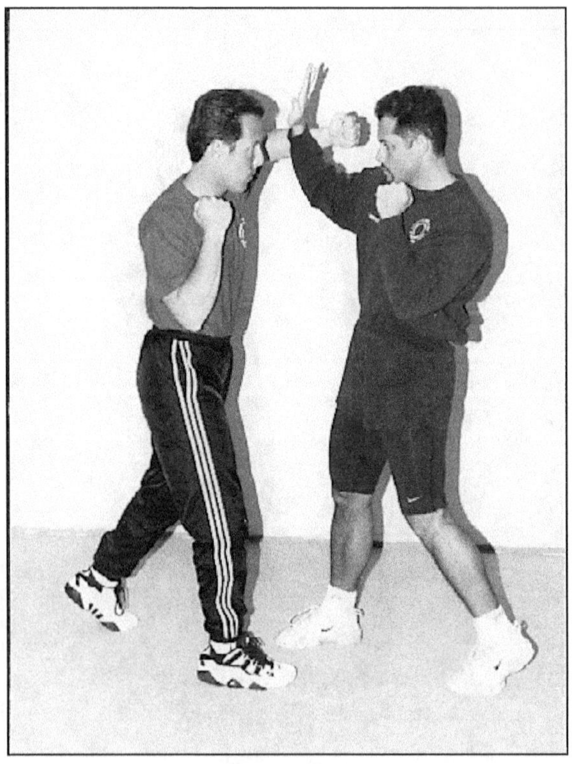

The mid block.

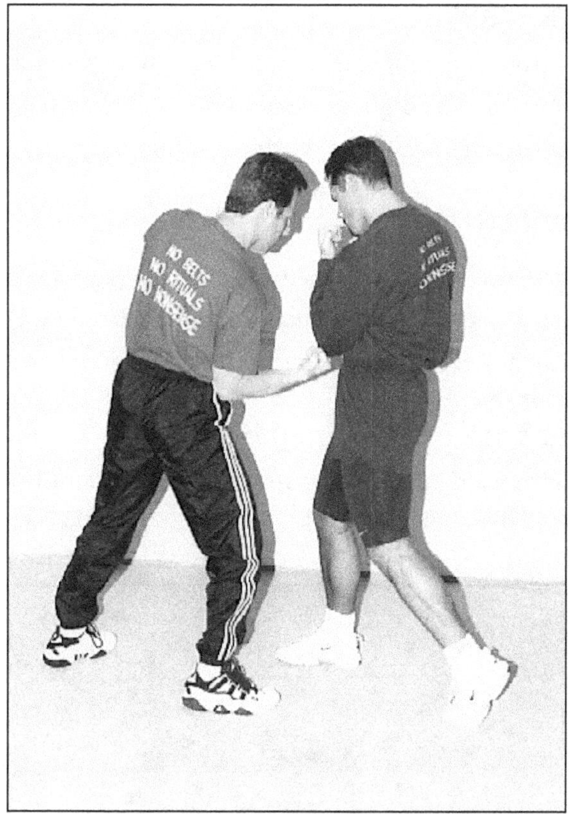

The elbow block.

Slipping

Slipping is a quick defensive maneuver that permits you to avoid an assailant's linear blow (e.g., jab, rear cross) without stepping out of range. Safe and effective slipping requires precise timing and is accomplished by quickly snapping the head and upper torso sideways (right or left) or backward to avoid the oncoming blow. One of the greatest advantages to slipping is that it frees your hands so that you can simultaneously counter your attacker. There are three ways to slip: right, left, and back.

Slipping Right

Begin from a fighting stance and quickly sway your head and upper torso to the right to avoid the assailant's blow. Quickly counterpunch or return to the starting position.

Slipping Left

Start from a fighting stance and quickly sway your head and upper torso to the left to avoid the assailant's linear blow. Quickly counterpunch or return to the starting position.

Slipping Back (or the Snap Back)

Begin from a fighting stance and quickly snap your head back enough to avoid being hit. Quickly counter or return to the starting position.

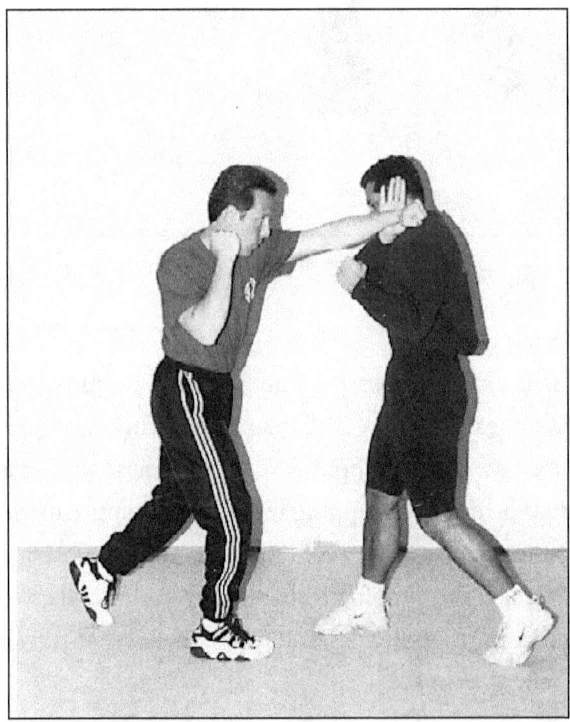

Pictured here, the horizontal parry.

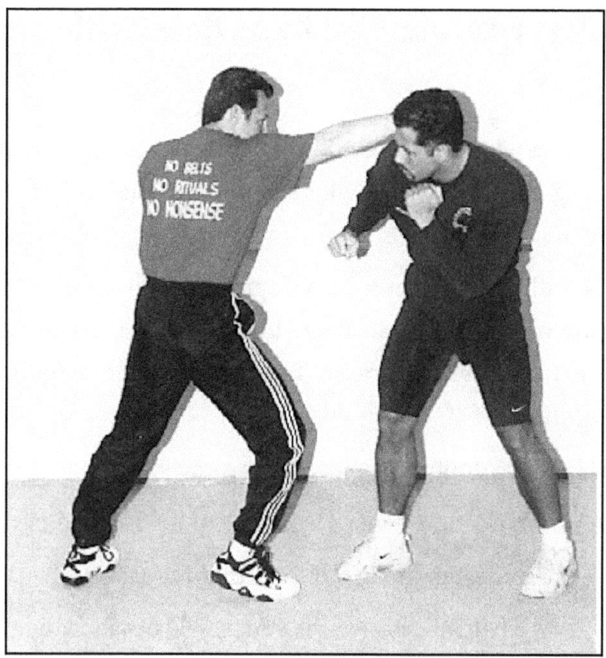

Slipping requires precise timing.

Footwork

The final component of defense is footwork. In defense, footwork allows you to disengage quickly from the range of attack and quickly re-engage with an effective counterattack. (For more information about footwork skills, see chapter 3.)

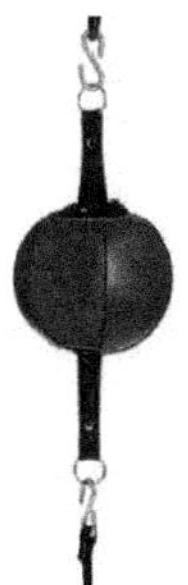

The best tool for developing defensive footwork is a full-length mirror.

Sidestep Double End bag Drill (with a partner)

Now that we covered all of the defensive techniques it's time to teach you a few defensive oriented double end bag drills. Let's start with the sidestep drill.

This drill is important for developing evasion skills and for enhancing your sense of range and timing. You'll need a training partner to perform this exercise. To perform the sidestepping drill, do the following:

1. Face the double end bag and assume a stance.
2. Your training partner grabs hold of the bag and pulls it back.
3. At the ideal moment, your partner releases the bag.
4. As the bag moves towards you, quickly evade it by sidestepping. For example, if you're standing in a southpaw stance, quickly step with your right foot to the right and move your left leg an equal distance. If you're standing in an orthodox stance, quickly step with your left foot to the left and have your right leg follow an equal distance. When performed correctly, the double end bag should miss you.
5. Then, deliver one rapid-fire combination on the bag.
6. Next, your training partner gains control of the swinging bag and you repeat the drill.
7. Perform the drill for a minimum of three rounds. Each round can last anywhere from two to five minutes.

Sidestep Double End bag Drill (solo practice)

This is a variation of the sidestep partner drill. Once again, this defensive exercise develops both footwork and timing skills. To perform the exercise, employ the following steps:

1. Face the double end bag and assume a fighting stance.
2. Begin throwing punching combinations at the bag.
3. After you complete a few combinations, quickly sidestep. If you're standing in a southpaw stance, quickly step with your right foot to the right and have your left leg follow an equal distance. If you're standing in an orthodox stance, quickly step with your left foot to the left and have your right leg follow an equal distance. When performed correctly, the bag should miss you.
4. Reposition yourself and resume throwing combinations at the swinging bag.
5. Perform the drill for a minimum of three rounds. Each round can last anywhere from two to five minutes.

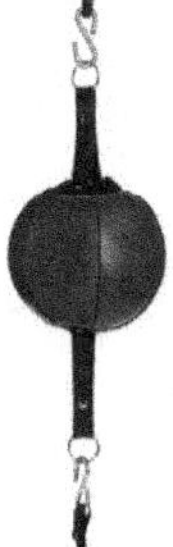

In order to gain maximum benefit from these defensive drills, you'll need to visualize the double end bag as a menacing opponent.

Circling Double End bag Drill (with a partner)

This circling drill is another defensive exercise that develops both footwork and quick counterpunching skills. Once again, you'll need a training partner to perform this exercise. To practice the circling drill, employ the following steps:

1. Face the double end bag and assume a fighting stance.
2. Your training partner grabs hold of the bag and pulls it back.
3. At the ideal moment, your partner releases the bag.
4. As the bag moves towards you, quickly circle away from it. For example, if you're standing in a southpaw stance, quickly step eight to twelve inches to the right with your right foot, and then use your right leg as a pivot point and wheel your entire rear leg to the right until the correct stance and positioning are acquired. If you're standing in an orthodox stance, quickly step eight to twelve inches to the left with your left foot and then use your left leg as a pivot point and wheel your entire rear leg to the left until the correct stance and positioning are acquired. When performed correctly, the double end bag should miss you.
5. While circling, simultaneously counterpunch bag. (The punch you choose will be dependent on a few factors, such as the distance of the target and angle of your body.)
6. Next, your training partner gains control of the swinging bag and you repeat the exercise.
7. Perform the drill for a minimum of three rounds. Each round can last anywhere from two to five minutes.

Circling Double End bag Drill (solo practice)

This is a variation of the partner drill. To perform the exercise, employ the following steps:

1. Face the double end bag and assume a fighting stance.
2. Begin throwing combinations at the bag.
3. After you complete a few combinations, circle away from from the returning bag. If you're standing in a right (southpaw) stance, quickly step eight to twelve inches to the right with your right foot, and then use your right leg as a pivot point and wheel your entire rear leg to the right until the correct stance and positioning are acquired. If you're standing in a left (orthodox) stance, quickly step eight to twelve inches to the left with your left foot and then use your left leg as a pivot point and wheel your entire rear leg to the left until the correct stance and positioning are acquired. When performed correctly, the bag should miss you.
4. While circling, simultaneously counterpunch the bag. Again, the punch you choose will be dependent on the distance of the bag and angle of your body.
5. Perform the drill for a minimum of three rounds. Each round can last anywhere from two to five minutes.

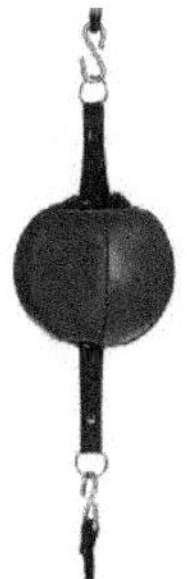

Don't forget! You can significantly reduce defensive reaction time by applying some of the following strategies: (1) Recognize advance information about your opponent's attack. (2) Limit your number of defensive options to a particular attack. (3) Make your defensive response natural and simple. (4) Practice, practice, practice!

Slipping Double End Bag Drill (with a partner)

This is another defensive drill that works on both your slipping and snapback skills. To perform the exercise, employ the following steps:

1. Face the double end bag and assume a fighting stance.
2. Your training partner grabs hold of the bag and pulls it back.
3. At the ideal moment, your partner releases the bag.
4. As the bag moves towards you, slip your head and body to the side. Try to visualize the opponent's punch coming at you. Remember, it's important that your mental images are clear, strong, and consistent.
5. Next, your training partner gains control of the swinging bag and you repeat the exercise.
6. Perform the drill for a minimum of three rounds. Each round can last anywhere from two to five minutes.
7. To increase the level of difficulty of this drill, you can perform the slipping movements with your hands behind your back.

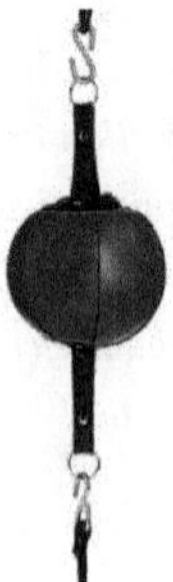

Slipping can be performed while simultaneously counter punching the opponent. It can also be used in conjunction with parring.

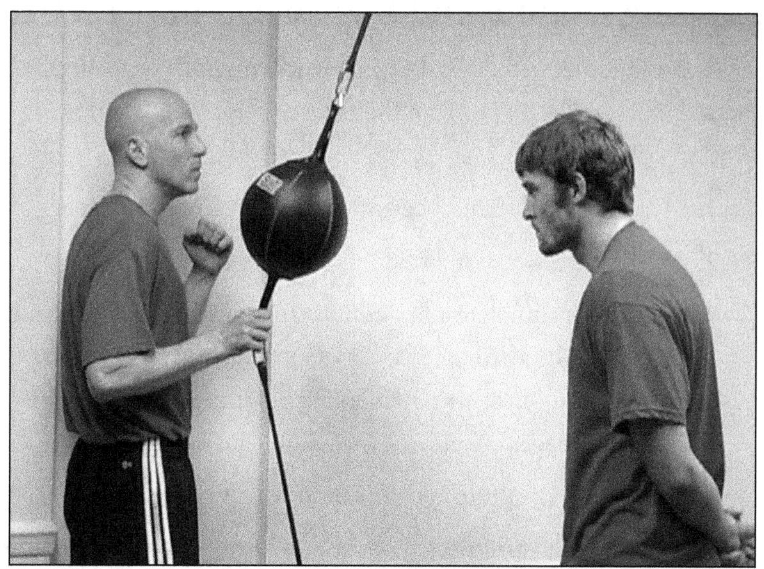

When performing the slipping drill (with a partner), be certain you are standing relatively close to the double end bag.

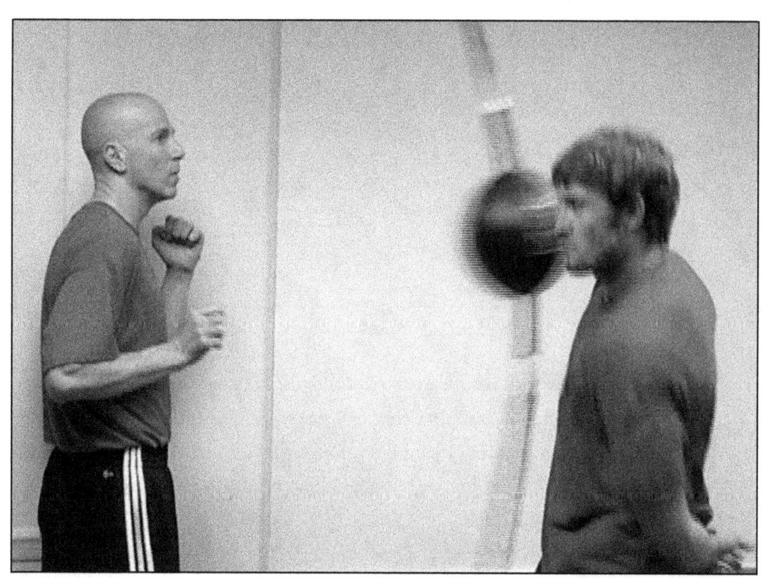

Remember to bend at the waist to safely clear your head from the rebounding bag.

Slipping Double End Bag Drill (solo practice)

This is another defensive drill that works on both your slipping and snapback skills. To perform the exercise, employ the following steps:

1. Face the double end bag and assume a fighting stance.
2. Begin throwing combinations at the bag.
3. After you complete a few combinations, arbitrarily slip your head and body to the side. Try to visualize the opponent's punch coming at you. Remember, it's important that your mental images are clear, strong, and consistent.
4. Return to the stance position and resume punching.
5. Perform the drill for a minimum of three rounds. Each round can last anywhere from two to five minutes.

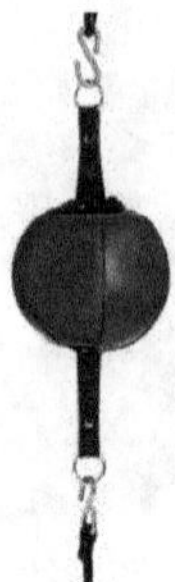

Defensive competency requires you to be adequately prepared to defend against a myriad of adversaries, including poorly skilled opponents. For example, you must be capable of defending against a tight boxer's hook as well as a sloppy, awkward haymaker.

Sidestep Drill Workout Routines (with a partner)

Skill Level	Duration of Each Round	Rest Period	Total Number of rounds
Beginner	1 minute	2 minutes	3
Beginner	1 minute	1 minute	3
Beginner	2 minutes	2 minutes	3
Beginner	2 minutes	1 minute	3
Intermediate	3 minutes	2 minutes	5
Intermediate	3 minutes	1 minute	5
Intermediate	3 minutes	2 minutes	6
Intermediate	3 minutes	1 minute	6
Advanced	4 minutes	2 minutes	8
Advanced	4 minutes	1 minute	8
Advanced	5 minutes	2 minutes	10
Advanced	5 minutes	1 minute	10

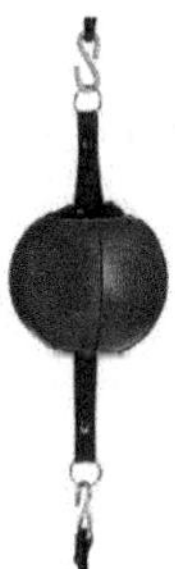

Rope skipping is another effective way of improving your footwork skills. It can be performed as an independent workout or added to your double end bag routine. Please see the section on interval training for more information.

Sidestep Drill Workout Routines (solo training)

Skill Level	Duration of Each Round	Rest Period	Total Number of rounds
Beginner	1 minute	2 minutes	3
Beginner	1 minute	1 minute	3
Beginner	2 minutes	2 minutes	3
Beginner	2 minutes	1 minute	3
Intermediate	3 minutes	2 minutes	5
Intermediate	3 minutes	1 minute	5
Intermediate	3 minutes	2 minutes	6
Intermediate	3 minutes	1 minute	6
Advanced	4 minutes	2 minutes	8
Advanced	4 minutes	1 minute	8
Advanced	5 minutes	2 minutes	10
Advanced	5 minutes	1 minute	10

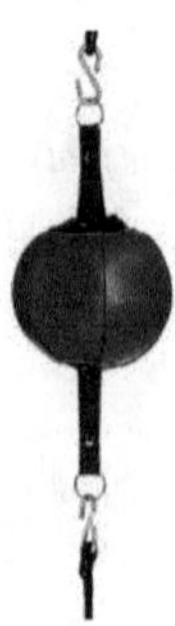

A good defensive structure is predicated on a stance that minimizes target exposure, facilitates balance and mobility, and permits quick and evasive movement.

Circling Drill Workout Routines (with a partner)

Skill Level	Duration of Each Round	Rest Period	Total Number of rounds
Beginner	1 minute	2 minutes	3
Beginner	1 minute	1 minute	3
Beginner	2 minutes	2 minutes	3
Beginner	2 minutes	1 minute	3
Intermediate	3 minutes	2 minutes	5
Intermediate	3 minutes	1 minute	5
Intermediate	3 minutes	2 minutes	6
Intermediate	3 minutes	1 minute	6
Advanced	4 minutes	2 minutes	8
Advanced	4 minutes	1 minute	8
Advanced	5 minutes	2 minutes	10
Advanced	5 minutes	1 minute	10

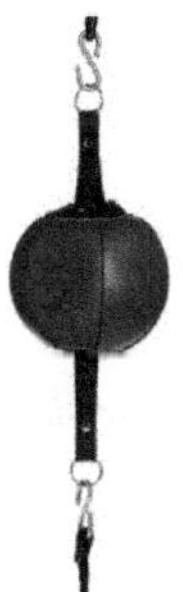

Ideally, your best defense is a strong and powerful offense, but in reality there will be situations and circumstances that demand a defensive response. However, don't misunderstand the necessity of a strong defense by becoming a defensive fighter. A defensive fighter is one who lets his assailant seize and maintain offensive control.

Circling Drill Workout Routines (solo training)			
Skill Level	**Duration of Each Round**	**Rest Period**	**Total Number of rounds**
Beginner	1 minute	2 minutes	3
Beginner	1 minute	1 minute	3
Beginner	2 minutes	2 minutes	3
Beginner	2 minutes	1 minute	3
Intermediate	3 minutes	2 minutes	5
Intermediate	3 minutes	1 minute	5
Intermediate	3 minutes	2 minutes	6
Intermediate	3 minutes	1 minute	6
Advanced	4 minutes	2 minutes	8
Advanced	4 minutes	1 minute	8
Advanced	5 minutes	2 minutes	10
Advanced	5 minutes	1 minute	10

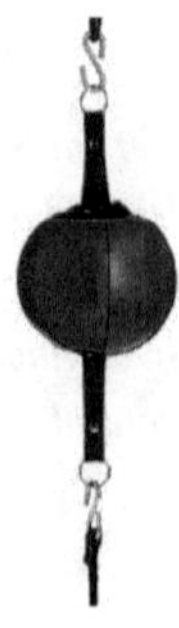

When working out on the bag, always be aware of your chin placement. Remember to always keep your chin angled slightly down. This makes you a more elusive target and help minimize direct strikes to your chin and nose. However, avoid forcing your chin down too low. This will inhibit the fluidity of your punches and ultimately slow you down.

Slipping Drill Workout Routines (solo training)

Skill Level	Duration of Each Round	Rest Period	Total Number of rounds
Beginner	1 minute	2 minutes	3
Beginner	1 minute	1 minute	3
Beginner	2 minutes	2 minutes	3
Beginner	2 minutes	1 minute	3
Intermediate	3 minutes	2 minutes	5
Intermediate	3 minutes	1 minute	5
Intermediate	3 minutes	2 minutes	6
Intermediate	3 minutes	1 minute	6
Advanced	4 minutes	2 minutes	8
Advanced	4 minutes	1 minute	8
Advanced	5 minutes	2 minutes	10
Advanced	5 minutes	1 minute	10

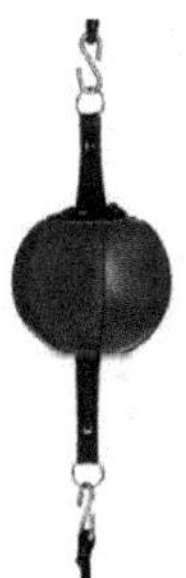

If you are training strictly for boxing, you can also add ducking or bobbing and weaving to your defensive double end bag training. Simply replace slipping maneuvers with a duck, bob or weave.

Workout Routine #9
Interval Training

Double end bag interval training requires you to alternate between two different activities throughout your workout. For our purposes, we are going to integrate five different activities with the double end bag. They are:

1. Rope skipping
2. Shadowboxing
3. Heavy bag training
4. Focus mitt training
5. Speed bag training

Rope Skipping Integration

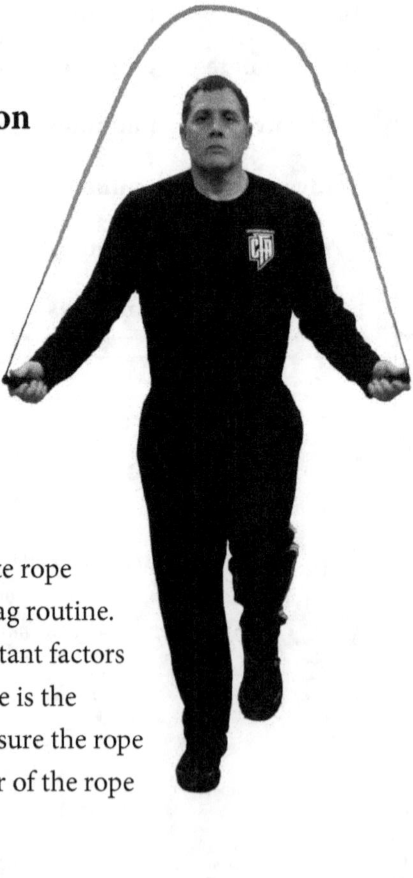

If you want to be quick and light on your feet, you will need to jump rope on a regular basis. Jumping rope is also one of the most effective ways of conditioning your heart and improving coordination, endurance, balance, agility, and body composition.

Fortunately, you can integrate rope skipping into your double end bag routine. However, one of the most important factors to consider when selecting a rope is the length. A simple method to measure the rope properly is to stand on the center of the rope with one foot. The handles of the rope should reach your armpits.

Interval training with the jump rope requires you to alternate exercises after every round. For example, your first round would include double end bag training, followed by a round of skipping rope, then double end bag training, and so on.

Here are some interval workout routines featuring double end bag training and rope skipping. For your convenience, I have included beginner, intermediate, and advanced workout programs.

Beginner Level
Interval Workout Routine (Skipping Rope)

Round	Activity	Duration of Each Round	Rest Period
1	Double End Bag	1 minute	2 minutes
2	Jump Rope	2 minutes	1 minute
3	Double End Bag	2 minutes	2 minutes
4	Jump Rope	1 minute	1 minute
5	Double End Bag	2 minutes	2 minutes
6	Jump Rope	2 minutes	1 minute
7	Double End Bag	1 minute	2 minutes
8	Jump Rope	1 minute	1 minute

Intermediate Level
Interval Workout Routine (Skipping Rope)

Round	Activity	Duration of Each Round	Rest Period
1	Double End Bag	2 minutes	2 minutes
2	Jump Rope	2 minutes	1 minute
3	Double End Bag	2 minutes	2 minutes
4	Jump Rope	2 minutes	1 minute
5	Double End Bag	2 minutes	2 minutes
6	Jump Rope	2 minutes	1 minute
7	Double End Bag	2 minutes	2 minutes
8	Jump Rope	2 minutes	1 minute
9	Double End Bag	2 minutes	2 minutes
10	Jump Rope	2 minutes	2 minutes

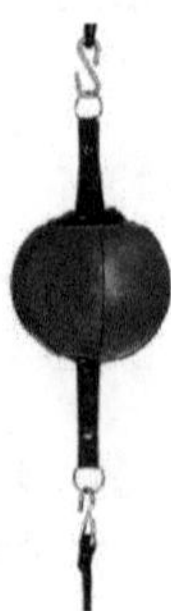

When moving around the double end bag, try to maintain a 50-percent weight distribution. This "noncommittal" weight distribution will provide you with the ability to move in any direction quickly and efficiently, while also supplying you with the necessary stability to withstand and defend against various blows.

Advanced Level
Interval Workout Routine (Skipping Rope)

Round	Activity	Duration of Each Round	Rest Period
1	Double End Bag	2 minutes	2 minutes
2	Jump Rope	2 minutes	1 minute
3	Double End Bag	3 minutes	2 minutes
4	Jump Rope	3 minutes	1 minute
5	Double End Bag	3 minutes	2 minutes
6	Jump Rope	3 minutes	1 minute
7	Double End Bag	3 minutes	2 minutes
8	Jump Rope	3 minutes	1 minute
9	Double End Bag	3 minutes	2 minutes
10	Jump Rope	3 minutes	2 minutes
11	Double End Bag	3 minutes	2 minutes
12	Jump Rope	3 minutes	2 minutes

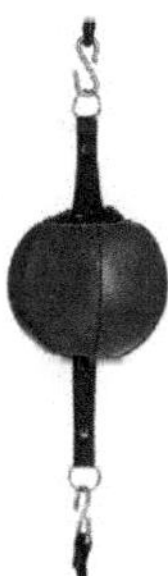

Learning how to skip rope can be very frustrating. Learn to be patient and the skill will come to you. It just takes time!

Rope Skipping Guidelines

Here are some other guidelines that will help you when skipping rope:

1. Relax your arms and shoulders when jumping.
2. Push off your toes and land gently on the balls of your feet.
3. Use your wrists and forearms to turn the rope, not your shoulders.
4. Maintain good posture and bend naturally at the knees and hips.
5. Jump low, approximately one inch off the ground.
6. Keep your head up and avoid the tendency to look down at your feet.
7. Keep both elbows close to your sides.
8. Avoid jumping rope barefoot.
9. Don't get frustrated by a tangled rope, it's part of the learning process.
10. Jump to different types of music and discover what tunes work best for you.

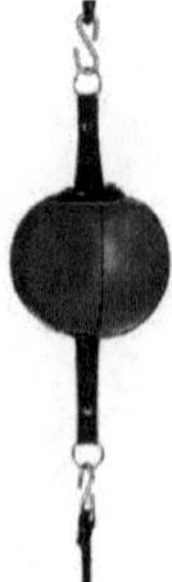

If you're not careful, you can develop shin splints from skipping rope on hard surfaces like concrete and asphalt. If possible, try to jump rope on a flexible surface like a rubber mat.

Shadowboxing Integration

Shadowboxing is the creative deployment of offensive and defensive techniques and maneuvers against an imaginary opponent. It requires intense mental concentration, honest self-analysis, and a deep commitment to improve.

For someone on a tight budget, the good news is that shadowboxing is inexpensive. All you need is a full-length mirror and a place to work out. The mirror is vital. It functions as a critic, your personal instructor. If you're honest, the mirror will be too. It will point out every mistake - telegraphing, sloppy footwork, poor body mechanics, and even lack of physical conditioning.

Proper shadowboxing develops speed, power, balance, footwork, combination skills, sound form, and finesse. It even promotes a better understanding of the ranges of combat.

As you progress, you can incorporate light dumbbells into shadowboxing workouts to enhance power and speed. Start off with one to three pounds and gradually work your way up.

Once again, interval training with shadowboxing requires you to alternate drills after every round. For example, your first round would include double end bag training, followed by a round of shadowboxing, then double end bag training, and so on.

What follows are a few interval workout routines featuring double end bag training and shadowboxing.

Beginner Level
Interval Workout Routine (Shadowboxing)

Round	Activity	Duration of Each Round	Rest Period
1	Double End Bag	1 minute	2 minutes
2	Shadowboxing	2 minutes	1 minute
3	Double End Bag	2 minutes	2 minutes
4	Shadowboxing	1 minute	1 minute
5	Double End Bag	2 minutes	2 minutes
6	Shadowboxing	2 minutes	1 minute
7	Double End Bag	1 minute	2 minutes
8	Shadowboxing	1 minute	1 minute

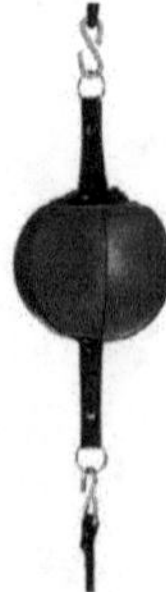

One of the most important elements of bag training is stability. If stability is compromised, then so is your stance. Here are three principles to keep in mind when trying to achieve stability in your stance: (1) keeping your center of gravity directly over your feet, (2) the lower you drop your center of gravity to its support base, the greater stability you will have, (3) the wider your stance, the greater your stability.

Intermediate Level
Interval Workout Routine (Shadowboxing)

Round	Activity	Duration of Each Round	Rest Period
1	Double End Bag	2 minutes	2 minutes
2	Shadowboxing	2 minutes	1 minute
3	Double End Bag	2 minutes	2 minutes
4	Shadowboxing	2 minutes	1 minute
5	Double End Bag	2 minutes	2 minutes
6	Shadowboxing	2 minutes	1 minute
7	Double End Bag	2 minutes	2 minutes
8	Shadowboxing	2 minutes	1 minute
9	Double End Bag	2 minutes	2 minutes
10	Shadowboxing	2 minutes	2 minutes

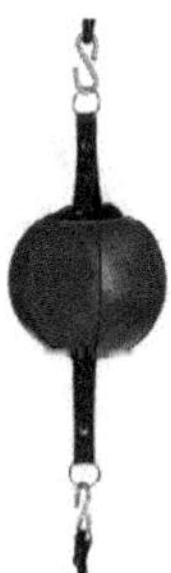

If you really want to challenge yourself, consider shadowboxing with a weight vest. This will strengthen your entire body, including your cardiovascular system.

Advanced Level
Interval Workout Routine (Shadowboxing)

Round	Activity	Duration of Each Round	Rest Period
1	Double End Bag	2 minutes	2 minutes
2	Shadowboxing	2 minutes	1 minute
3	Double End Bag	3 minutes	2 minutes
4	Shadowboxing	3 minutes	1 minute
5	Double End Bag	3 minutes	2 minutes
6	Shadowboxing	3 minutes	1 minute
7	Double End Bag	3 minutes	2 minutes
8	Shadowboxing	3 minutes	1 minute
9	Double End Bag	3 minutes	2 minutes
10	Shadowboxing	3 minutes	2 minutes
11	Double End Bag	3 minutes	2 minutes
12	Shadowboxing	3 minutes	2 minutes

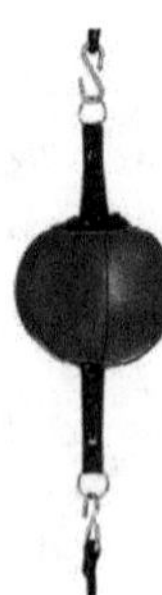

If you want to improve your punching power, you can use light dumbbells (1- 5 pounds) during your shadow fighting sessions.

Heavy Bag Integration

The heavy bag is a cylindrical shaped bag designed to be repeatedly kicked, punched and struck by the practitioner. Most traditional heavy bags are 14 inches in diameter and 42 inches in length.

The interior of the bag is usually filled with either cotton fiber, thick foam, sand or other durable material. The exterior of the heavy bag can be constructed with a variety of different materials including heavy canvas or vinyl while more expensive types are made of thick leather.

This unique piece of training equipment that provides a full range of benefits for the practitioner. Some include:

- **Developing and sharpening your fighting skills.**
- **Conditioning your entire body for the rigors of intense fighting.**
- **Improving muscular endurance.**
- **Strengthening your bones, tendons, and ligaments.**
- **Conditioning your cardiovascular system.**
- **Relieving stress and channeling aggressive energy in a productive manner.**
- **Developing several mental toughness attributes, such as instrumental aggression, immediate resilience, self-confidence, and attention control.**

Depending on the brand, heavy bags can weigh anywhere from seventy-five to two hundred and fifty pounds. However, the average bag will weigh approximately eighty-five pounds.

Here are a few interval workout routines featuring both the double end bag and the heavy bag.

Beginner Level
Interval Workout Routine (Heavy Bag)

Round	Activity	Duration of Each Round	Rest Period
1	Double End Bag	1 minute	2 minutes
2	Heavy Bag	2 minutes	1 minute
3	Double End Bag	2 minutes	2 minutes
4	Heavy Bag	1 minute	1 minute
5	Double End Bag	2 minutes	2 minutes
6	Heavy Bag	2 minutes	1 minute
7	Double End Bag	1 minute	2 minutes
8	Heavy Bag	1 minute	1 minute

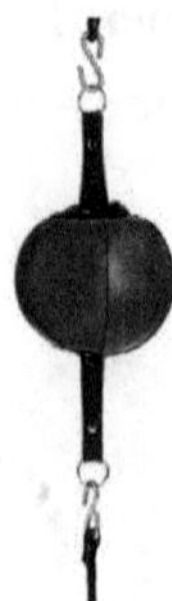

Did you know the legendary Bruce Lee used to work out on a 300-pound heavy bag.

Intermediate Level
Interval Workout Routine (Heavy Bag)

Round	Activity	Duration of Each Round	Rest Period
1	Double End Bag	2 minutes	2 minutes
2	Heavy Bag	2 minutes	1 minute
3	Double End Bag	2 minutes	2 minutes
4	Heavy Bag	2 minutes	1 minute
5	Double End Bag	2 minutes	2 minutes
6	Heavy Bag	2 minutes	1 minute
7	Double End Bag	2 minutes	2 minutes
8	Heavy Bag	2 minutes	1 minute
9	Double End Bag	2 minutes	2 minutes
10	Heavy Bag	2 minutes	2 minutes

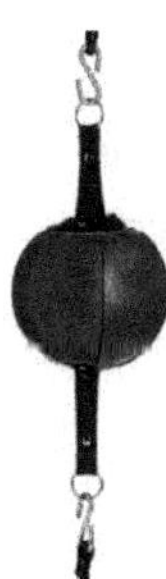

The Heavy Bag is not just limited to stand-up fighting. It can also be used for ground fighting strikes. This is often referred to as "ground and pound" techniques.

Advanced Level
Interval Workout Routine (Heavy Bag)

Round	Activity	Duration of Each Round	Rest Period
1	Double End Bag	2 minutes	2 minutes
2	Heavy Bag	2 minutes	1 minute
3	Double End Bag	3 minutes	2 minutes
4	Heavy Bag	3 minutes	1 minute
5	Double End Bag	3 minutes	2 minutes
6	Heavy Bag	3 minutes	1 minute
7	Double End Bag	3 minutes	2 minutes
8	Heavy Bag	3 minutes	1 minute
9	Double End Bag	3 minutes	2 minutes
10	Heavy Bag	3 minutes	2 minutes
11	Double End Bag	3 minutes	2 minutes
12	Heavy Bag	3 minutes	2 minutes

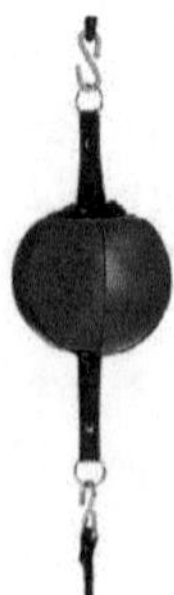

If you workout on the heavy bag with a significant amount of intensity, you can turn it into a challenging cardiovascular workout. However, this will require you to throw your punches, kicks and strikes at a very respectable pace.

Focus Mitt Integration

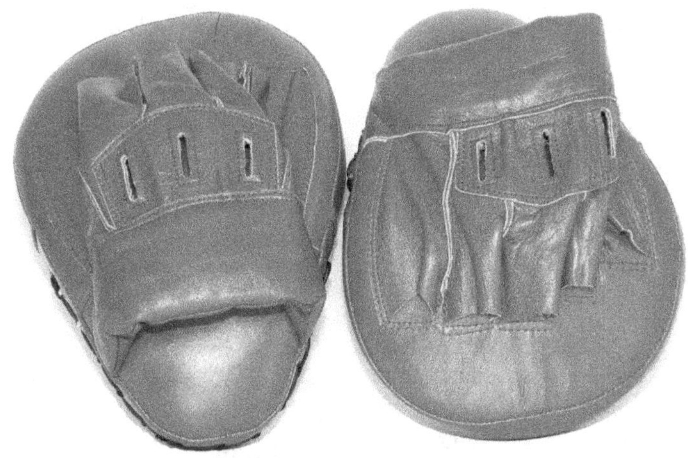

The focus mitt (or punching mitt) is an exceptional piece of equipment that can be used by just about anyone. It develops punching speed, rhythm, endurance, accuracy, timing, reflexes, footwork, punching combinations, and counterpunching techniques.

By placing the mitts at various angles and levels, you can perform every conceivable kick, punch, or strike know to man. Properly utilized, focus mitts will refine your defensive reaction time and condition your entire body.

Focus mitts are constructed of durable leather designed to withstand tremendous punishment. Compared to other pieces of training equipment, the focus mitt is relatively inexpensive. However, an effective workout requires two mitts (one for each hand). You will also need a training partner (called the feeder) to hold the mitts. Your partner plays a vital role during your workouts by determining which combinations you will throw and their speed of delivery. In fact, the intensity of your workouts will depend largely upon his or her ability to manipulate the mitts and push you to your limit.

Double End Bag Workout

To benefit from any focus-mitt workout, you must learn to concentrate intensely throughout the entire session. Block out all distractions. Try to visualize the mitt as a living, breathing opponent, not an inanimate target. This type of visualization will make all the difference in your training.

Here are few sample interval routines integrating the double end bag with the focus mitts.

Beginner Level
Interval Workout Routine (Focus Mitts)

Round	Activity	Duration of Each Round	Rest Period
1	Double End Bag	1 minute	2 minutes
2	Focus Mitts	2 minutes	1 minute
3	Double End Bag	2 minutes	2 minutes
4	Focus Mitts	1 minute	1 minute
5	Double End Bag	2 minutes	2 minutes
6	Focus Mitts	2 minutes	1 minute
7	Double End Bag	1 minute	2 minutes
8	Focus Mitts	1 minute	1 minute

Intermediate Level
Interval Workout Routine (Focus Mitts)

Round	Activity	Duration of Each Round	Rest Period
1	Double End Bag	2 minutes	2 minutes
2	Focus Mitts	2 minutes	1 minute
3	Double End Bag	2 minutes	2 minutes
4	Focus Mitts	2 minutes	1 minute
5	Double End Bag	2 minutes	2 minutes
6	Focus Mitts	2 minutes	1 minute
7	Double End Bag	2 minutes	2 minutes
8	Focus Mitts	2 minutes	1 minute
9	Double End Bag	2 minutes	2 minutes
10	Focus Mitts	2 minutes	2 minutes

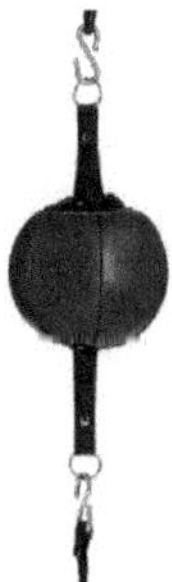

I frequently tell my students that a good focus mitt feeder is one step ahead of his training partner, whereas a great focus mitt feeder is two steps ahead of his partner.

Advanced Level
Interval Workout Routine (Focus Mitts)

Round	Activity	Duration of Each Round	Rest Period
1	Double End Bag	2 minutes	2 minutes
2	Focus Mitts	2 minutes	1 minute
3	Double End Bag	3 minutes	2 minutes
4	Focus Mitts	3 minutes	1 minute
5	Double End Bag	3 minutes	2 minutes
6	Focus Mitts	3 minutes	1 minute
7	Double End Bag	3 minutes	2 minutes
8	Focus Mitts	3 minutes	1 minute
9	Double End Bag	3 minutes	2 minutes
10	Focus Mitts	3 minutes	2 minutes
11	Double End Bag	3 minutes	2 minutes
12	Focus Mitts	3 minutes	2 minutes

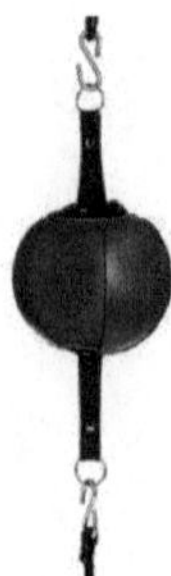

Focus mitt training also requires pinpoint accuracy. If you don't hit the mitt directly in the center, your punch will glance off the pad.

Speed Bag Integration

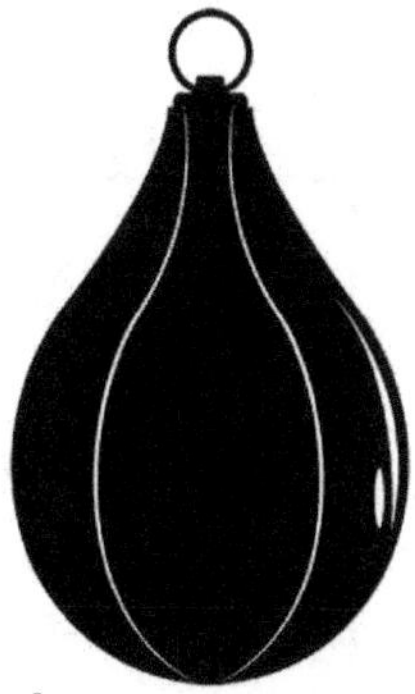

The speed is used by boxers to develop coord endurance, timing, and rhythm. However, let me the record and state that I'm not a big fan of the s bag. In fact, I believe it's an antiquated training tool that develops bad habits. Some include the following:

1. **Centerline exposure** - in order to strike t speed bag effectively, you must stand squarely in front of the bag. This means you must sacrifice your fighting stance and completely expose your centerline.
2. **Unrealistic attack rhythm** - the impact rhythm generated on a speed bag isn't remotely close to the attack rhythms used in real fighting.
3. **Improper fist positioning** - the speed bag requires you to ***roll*** your fists and strike it with the edge of your hands. If you would never punch this way in a real fight, then why on earth would you train this way?
4. **Poor body mechanics** - to maintain a fast striking rhythm on the bag, you must abandon proper punching mechanics.
5. **Mobility limitation** -since the speed bag is attached to a platform, your movement is significantly restricted. In fact, you must stay in close contact with the bag at all times.
6. **Lack of power** - to maintain the proper striking rhythm on the bag, you must only hit it with a slight amount of force. This style of punching is impractical for both the boxing ring and the street.

Nevertheless, I'm including the speed bag in this section out of respect for the boxing purist who insists on adding it to their training.

Beginner Level
Interval Workout Routine (Speed Bag)

Round	Activity	Duration of Each Round	Rest Period
1	Double End Bag	1 minute	2 minutes
2	Speed Bag	2 minutes	1 minute
3	Double End Bag	2 minutes	2 minutes
4	Speed Bag	1 minute	1 minute
5	Double End Bag	2 minutes	2 minutes
6	Speed Bag	2 minutes	1 minute
7	Double End Bag	1 minute	2 minutes
8	Speed Bag	1 minute	1 minute

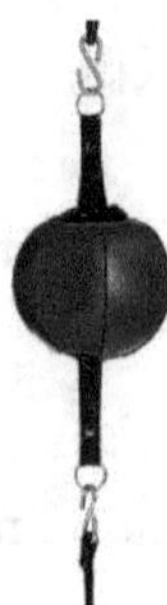

Proper breathing is one of the most important and often neglected aspects of bag work. Proper breathing promotes muscular relaxation and increases the speed and efficiency of your combinations. The rate at which you breathe will also determine how quickly your cardiorespiratory system can recover from a round.

Intermediate Level
Interval Workout Routine (Speed Bag)

Round	Activity	Duration of Each Round	Rest Period
1	Double End Bag	2 minutes	2 minutes
2	Speed Bag	2 minutes	1 minute
3	Double End Bag	2 minutes	2 minutes
4	Speed Bag	2 minutes	1 minute
5	Double End Bag	2 minutes	2 minutes
6	Speed Bag	2 minutes	1 minute
7	Double End Bag	2 minutes	2 minutes
8	Speed Bag	2 minutes	1 minute
9	Double End Bag	2 minutes	2 minutes
10	Speed Bag	2 minutes	2 minutes

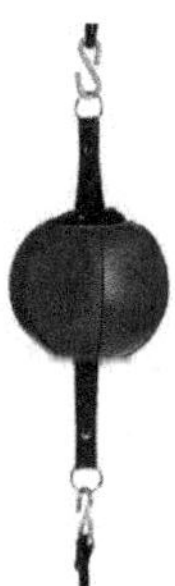

When it comes to preparing for the ring or the street, remember to train the way you want to fight and fight the way you train!

Advanced Level
Interval Workout Routine (Speed Bag)

Round	Activity	Duration of Each Round	Rest Period
1	Double End Bag	2 minutes	2 minutes
2	Speed Bag	2 minutes	1 minute
3	Double End Bag	3 minutes	2 minutes
4	Speed Bag	3 minutes	1 minute
5	Double End Bag	3 minutes	2 minutes
6	Speed Bag	3 minutes	1 minute
7	Double End Bag	3 minutes	2 minutes
8	Speed Bag	3 minutes	1 minute
9	Double End Bag	3 minutes	2 minutes
10	Speed Bag	3 minutes	2 minutes
11	Double End Bag	3 minutes	2 minutes
12	Speed Bag	3 minutes	2 minutes

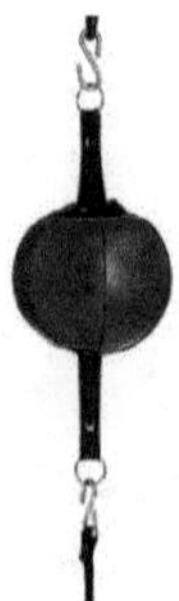

Remember to tighten your fists upon impact with bag. This action will allow your punches to travel with optimum speed and efficiency, and it will also augment the impact power of your strike.

Workout Routine #10
Bare-Knuckle Training

While bag gloves are essential for protecting your hands when training, every once in a while you should workout without them. In fact, this type of bare-knuckle training is critical to anyone interested in reality-based self-defense training.

As I have stated in many of my other books, in the streets you don't have the luxury of rules, regulations or protective equipment. You have to make due with what you have at the moment of a high-risk self-defense encounter. Bare-knuckle training will help prepare you for the real thing. In fact, striking the double end bag without hand protection is essential because it conditions your hands for the rigors of street fighting.

However, bare-knuckle bag training is very hard on your wrists, hands, and knuckles. Transitioning from hand protected training to bare-knuckles is not easy. Initially, punching bare-fisted will feel awkward to even the most experienced fighter. Therefore, it's imperative to start out with approximately 25% of you punching power and increase it over a period of time.

One of the best ways to condition your hands and wrists for bare-knuckle fighting is to practice my ***glove on/glove off*** program. Essentially, you are going to alternate between bare handed and gloved punching. After several months, you can progress to exclusively bare-knuckle training.

What follows are several ***glove on/glove off*** workout routines.

Beginner Level
Bare-Knuckle Training (Glove On/Glove Off)

Round	Activity	Duration of Each Round	Rest Period
1	Glove on	1 minute	2 minutes
2	Glove off	30 seconds	1 minute
3	Glove on	2 minutes	2 minutes
4	Glove off	45 seconds	1 minute
5	Glove on	2 minutes	2 minutes
6	Glove off	1 minute	1 minute
7	Glove on	2 minutes	2 minutes
8	Glove off	90 seconds	1 minute

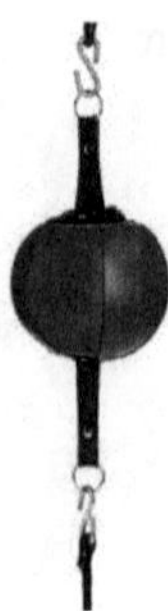

Bare-knuckle fighting is a skill set that's much different from boxing and other combat sports. In fact, I know of several stories where professional boxers have broken their hands during a bare handed fist fight. This is because most professional fighters don't condition their hands for this type of fighting.

Intermediate Level
Bare-Knuckle Training (Glove On/Glove Off)

Round	Activity	Duration of Each Round	Rest Period
1	Glove on	2 minutes	2 minutes
2	Glove off	1 minute	1 minute
3	Glove on	2 minutes	2 minutes
4	Glove off	90 seconds	1 minute
5	Glove on	2 minutes	2 minutes
6	Glove off	90 seconds	1 minute
7	Glove on	2 minutes	2 minutes
8	Glove off	2 minutes	1 minute
9	Glove on	2 minutes	2 minutes
10	Glove off	2 minutes	2 minutes

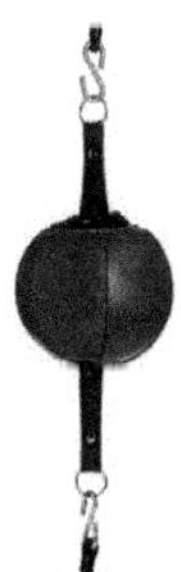

If bare-knuckle bag training is too hard on your hands, consider wearing hand wraps until your knuckles can handle it.

Advanced Level
Bare-Knuckle Training (Glove On/Glove Off)

Round	Activity	Duration of Each Round	Rest Period
1	Glove on	2 minutes	2 minutes
2	Glove off	2 minutes	1 minute
3	Glove on	3 minutes	2 minutes
4	Glove off	2 minutes	1 minute
5	Glove on	3 minutes	2 minutes
6	Glove off	2 1/2 minutes	1 minute
7	Glove on	3 minutes	2 minutes
8	Glove off	2 1/2 minutes	1 minute
9	Glove on	3 minutes	2 minutes
10	Glove off	3 minutes	2 minutes
11	Glove on	3 minutes	2 minutes
12	Glove off	3 minutes	2 minutes

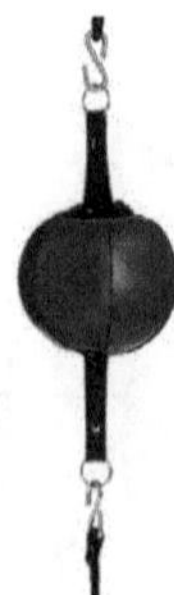

To avoid potential hand problems, don't perform bare-knuckle training more than five times per month.

Workout Routine #11
Impairment Training

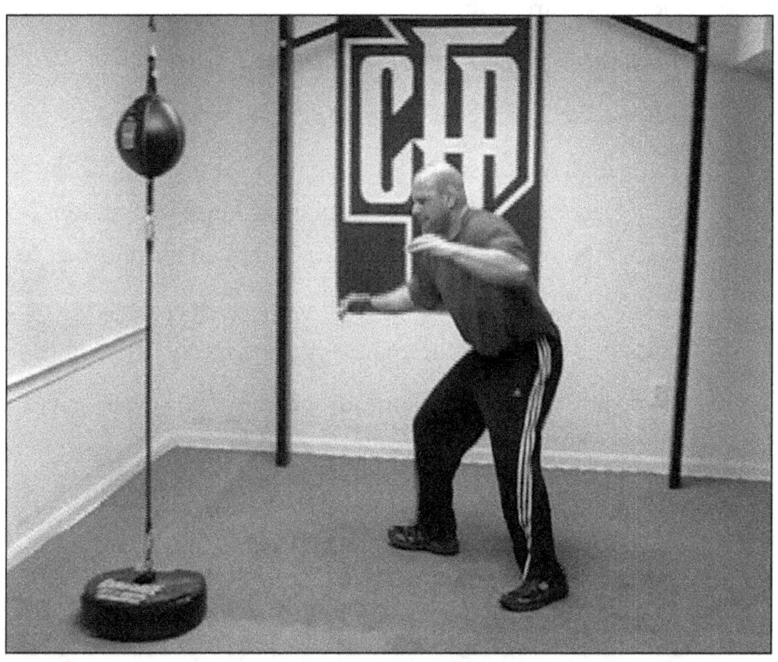

Impairment training teaches you how to fight when temporarily injured or impaired. There are several different types of impairment training routines you can perform on the double end bag. Let's take a look at one of them.

Disorientation Drill

The Disorientation drill replicates the lightheaded sensation you will feel when you get hit by the opponent. This exercise is particularly useful because it teaches you to continue fighting when you are dizzy and lose your balance during a fight. To perform the exercise, employ the following steps:

Double End Bag Workout

1. Start with both your hands at your sides and your head looking down at the floor.
2. Next, close your eyes and begin spinning your body in a clockwise direction.
3. Continue spinning for approximately 10 seconds.
4. After 10 seconds, your training partner calls out "fight!"
5. Immediately stop spinning, open your eyes and attack the double end bag with a barrage of punching combinations. Remember, you're going to be very dizzy, so do your best to maintain proper punching form.
6. Continue punching the bag for approximately 20 seconds.
7. Rest for a minimum of 5 minutes before going again.

Disorientation Drill Demonstration

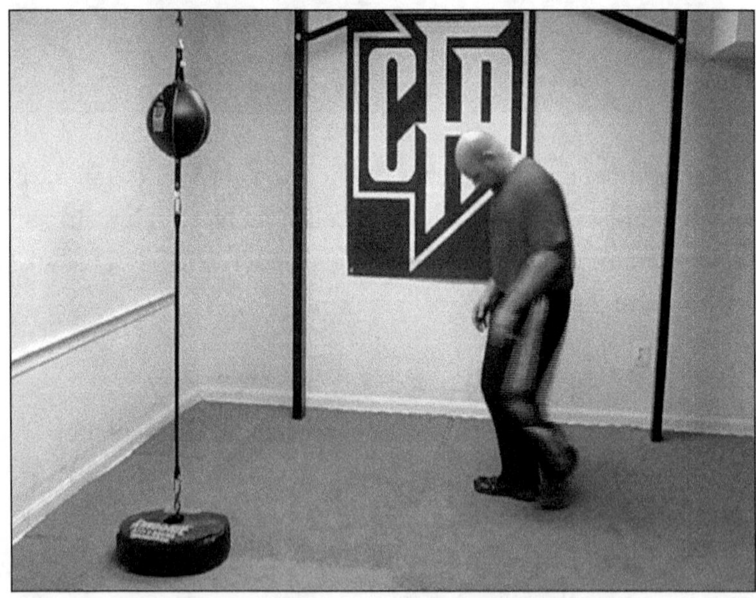

Step 1: The practitioner begins with his head down, eyes closed, and his arms at his sides.

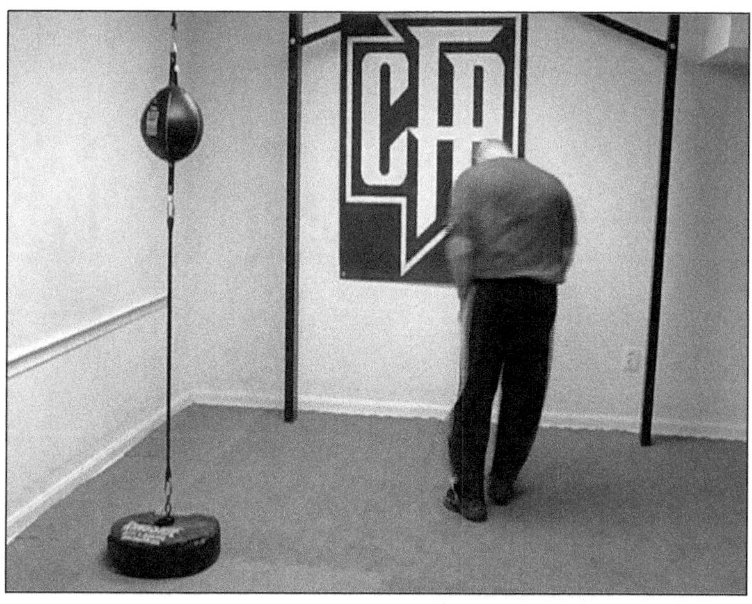

Step 2: The time keeper instructs him to begin spinning.

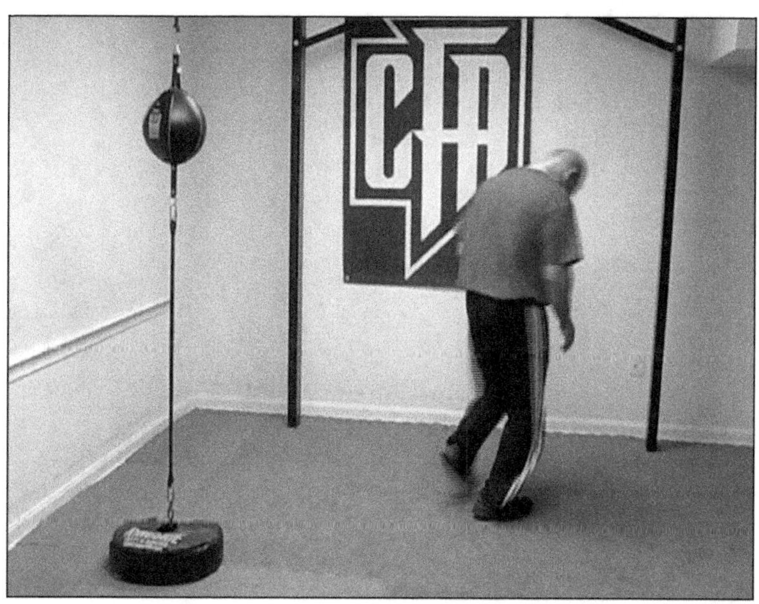

Step 3: The man spins his body in a clockwise direction.

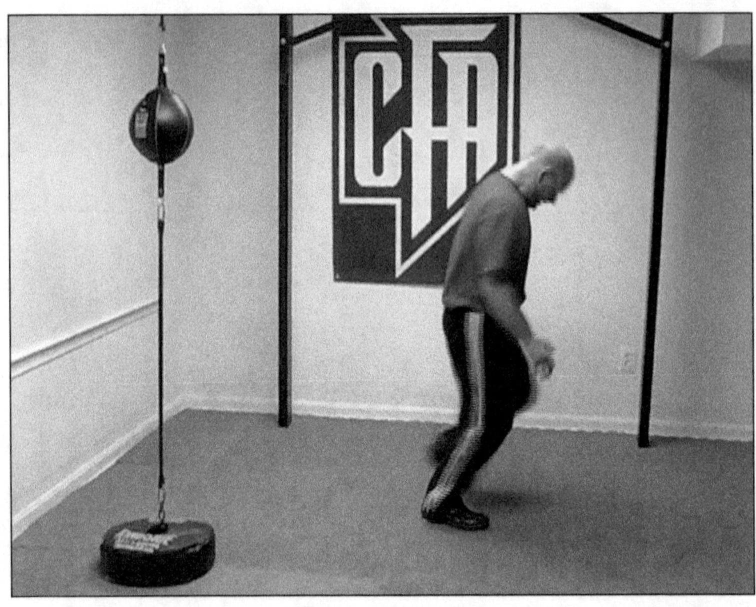

Step 4: He continues to spin with his eyes closed for approximately 10 seconds.

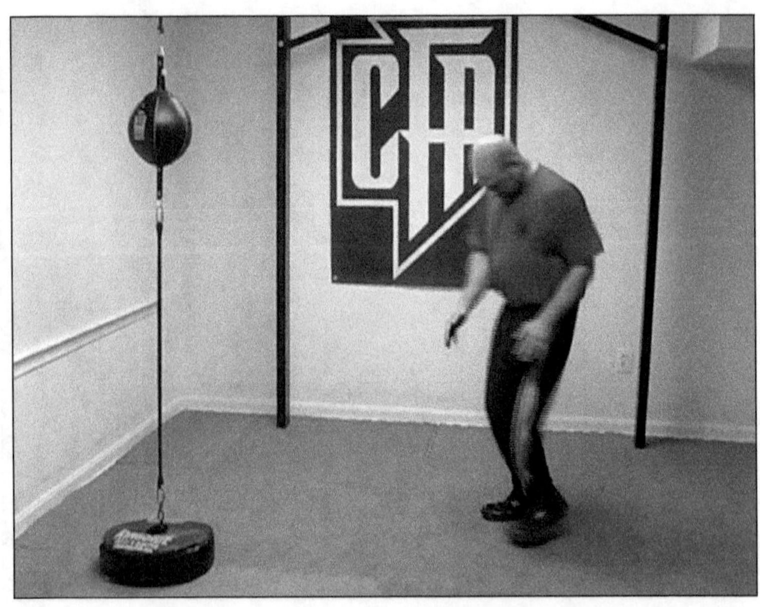

Step 5: At the end of 10 seconds, the time keeper yells, "fight!"

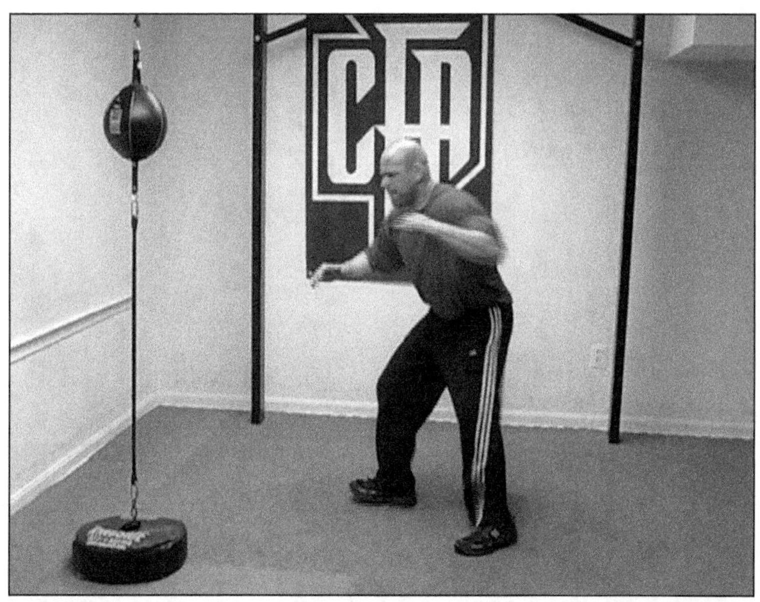

Step 6: The practitioner immediately opens his eyes and tries to balance himself.

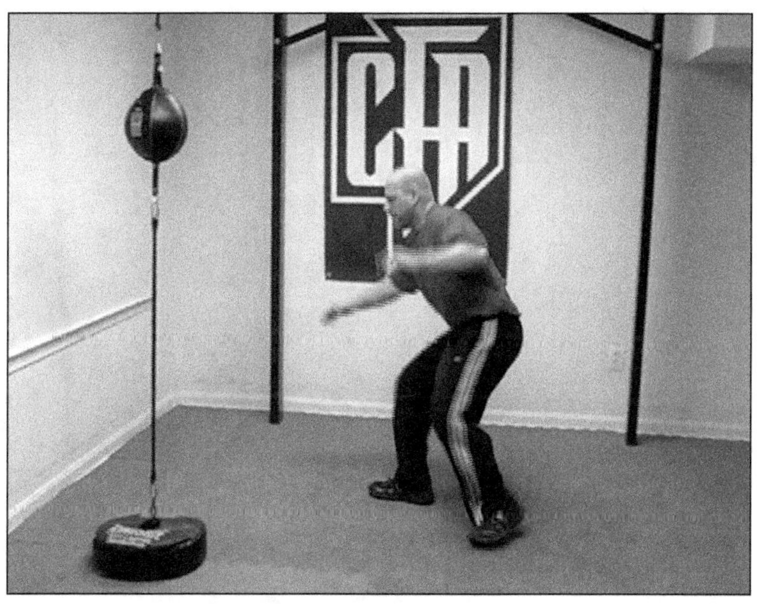

Step 7: The drill takes effect.

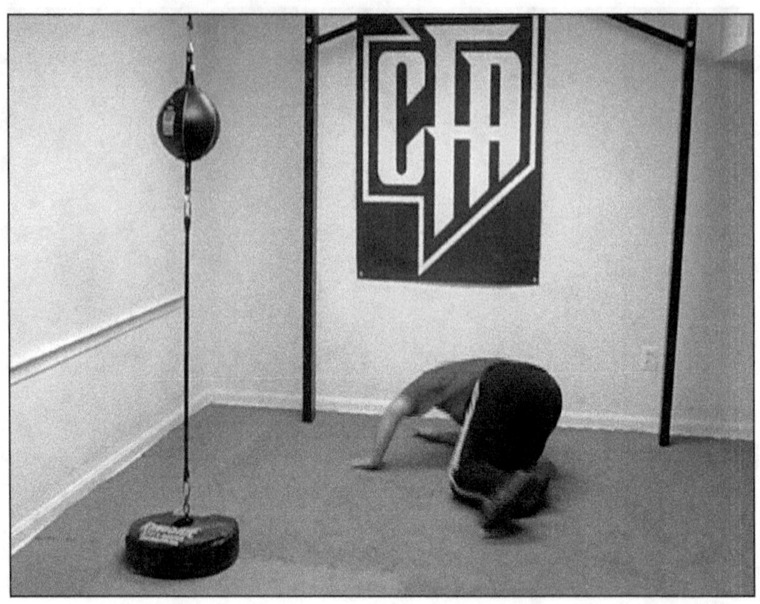

Step 8: The practitioner loses his balance and falls to the ground.

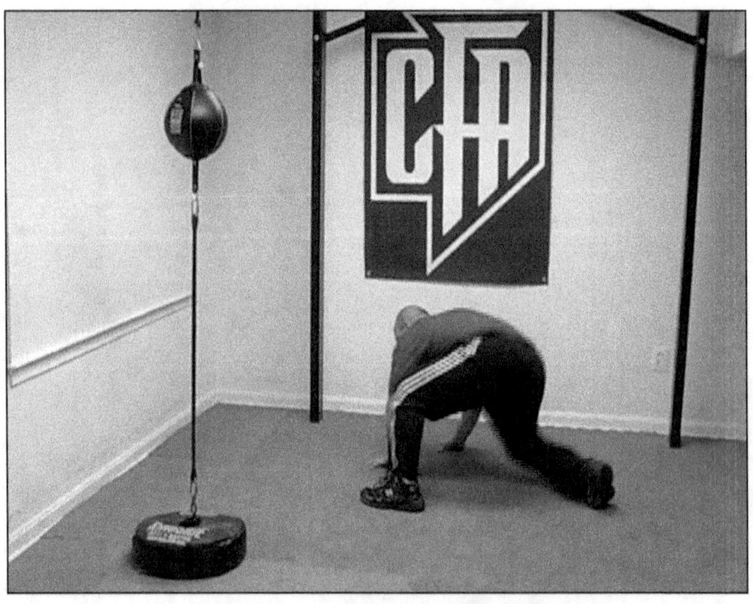

Step 9: He struggles to get back on his feet.

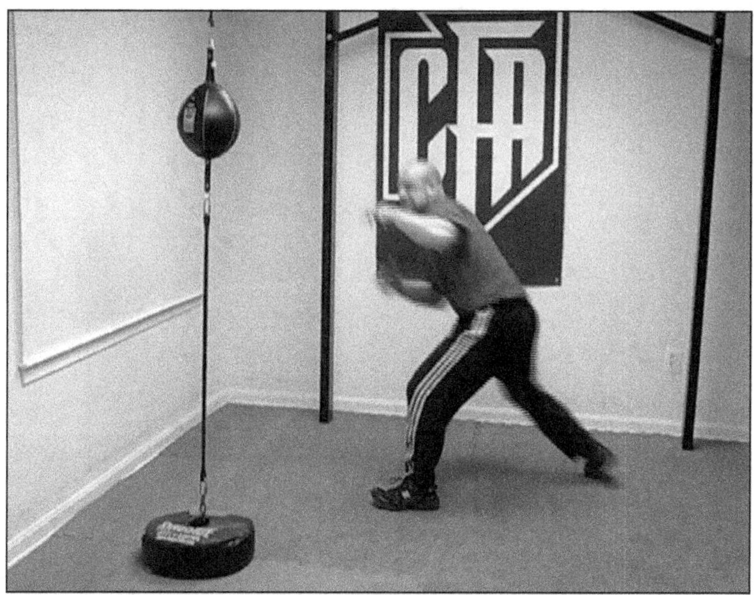

Step 10: He regains his balance and goes after the bag.

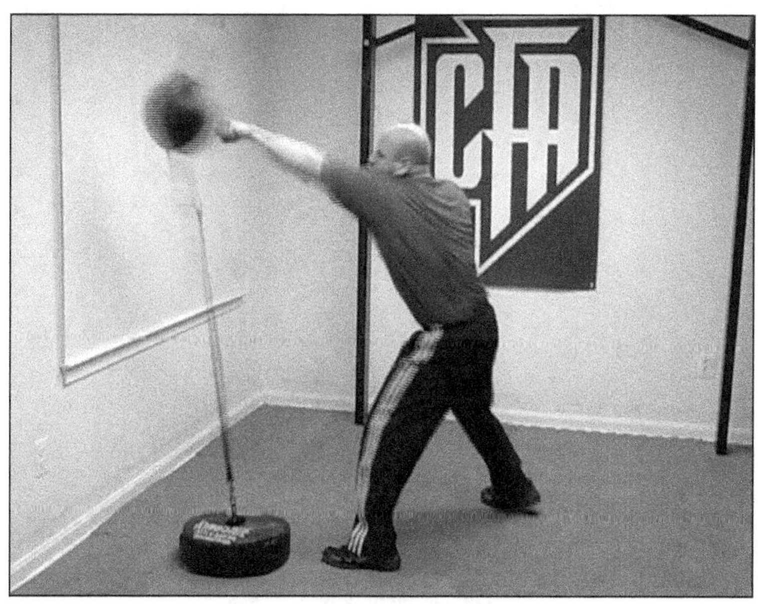

Step 11: He successfully lands his first blow.

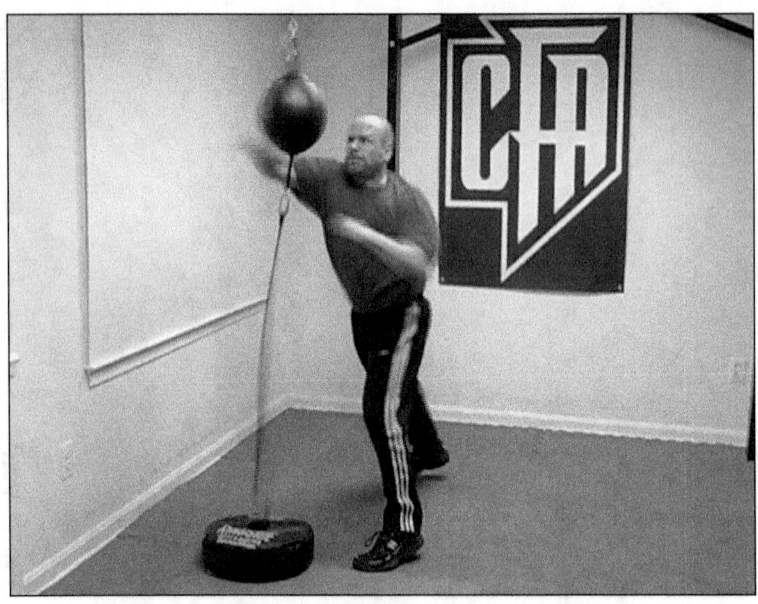

Step 12: His dizziness causes him to miss with his second punch.

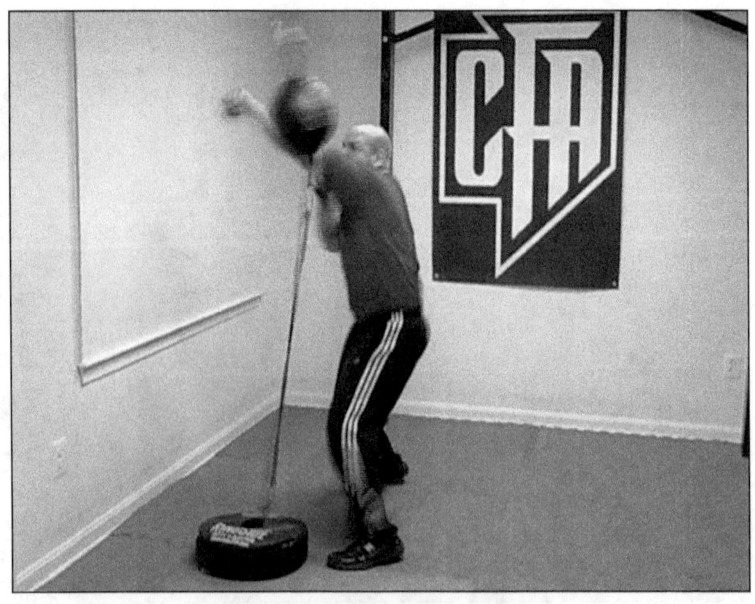

Step 13: He misses the target again.

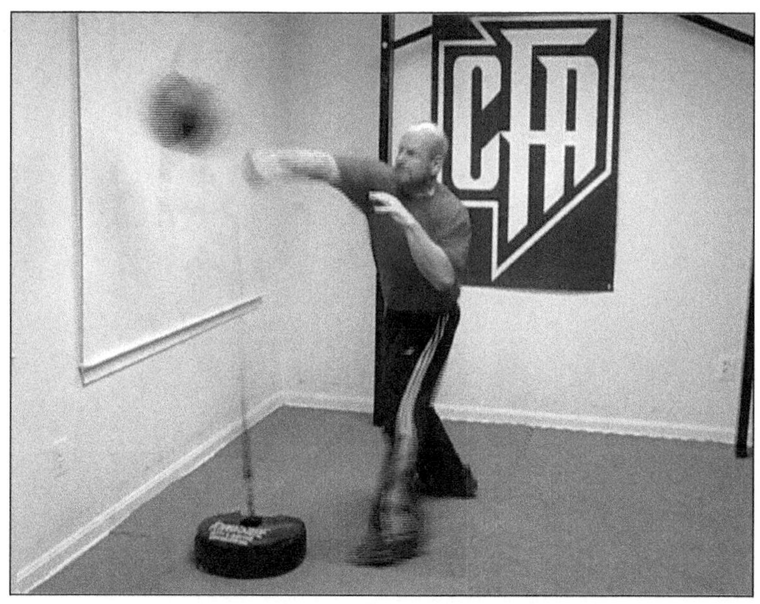

Step 14: His rear cross makes contact with the bag.

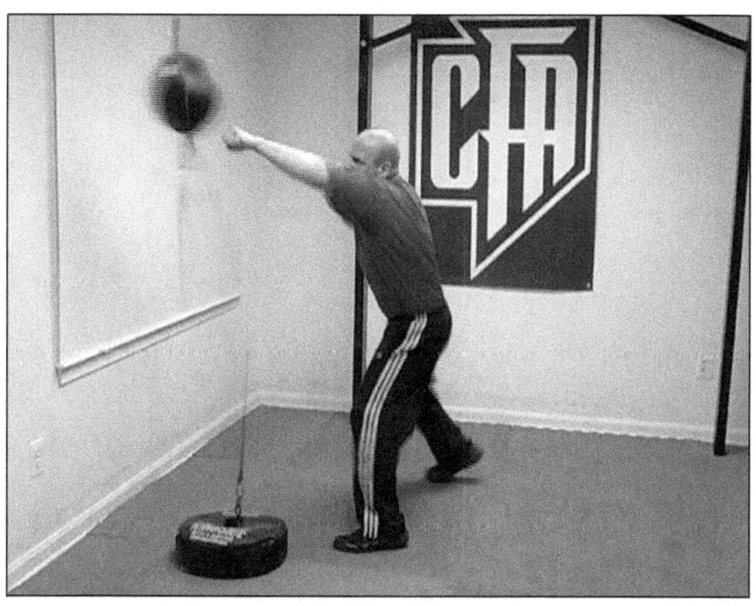

Step 15: Followed by a jab.

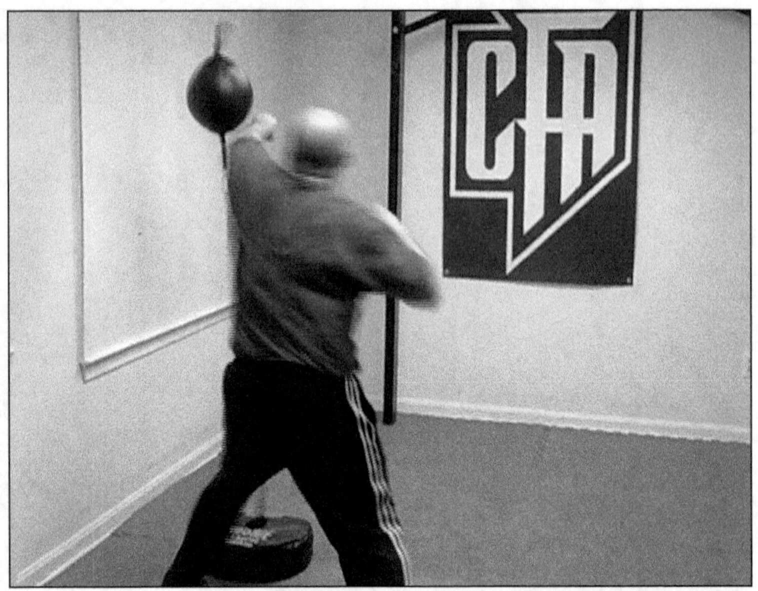

Step 16: He continues moving and hitting the bag for approximately 20 seconds.

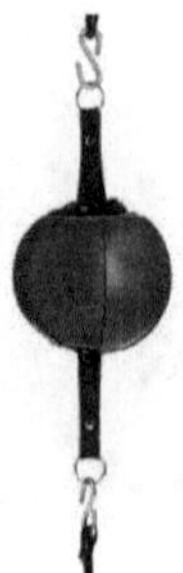

Be very careful when practicing the disorientation drill. Make certain your training area is away from windows, glass doors objects, children, and pets.

Disorientation Drill Workout Routines

Skill Level	Duration of Spin	Duration of Punching Round	Rest Period Between Rounds	Total Number of rounds
Beginner	5 seconds	10 seconds	10 minutes	2
Beginner	5 seconds	12 seconds	10 minutes	2
Beginner	8 seconds	14 seconds	10 minutes	2
Beginner	8 seconds	15 seconds	10 minutes	2
Intermediate	10 seconds	15 seconds	5 minutes	3
Intermediate	10 seconds	20 seconds	5 minutes	3
Intermediate	10 seconds	20 seconds	5 minutes	3
Intermediate	10 seconds	25 seconds	5 minutes	3
Advanced	10 seconds	25 seconds	5 minutes	4
Advanced	10 seconds	30 seconds	5 minutes	4
Advanced	10 seconds	45 seconds	5 minutes	4
Advanced	10 seconds	45 seconds	5 minutes	4

Other Impairment Drills

There are many other impairment drills that you can perform. Here are a few suggestions that will get you started.

1. Workout on the double end bag with one arm in a sling.
2. Wear an eye patch and see how it affects your punching skills.
3. Train when you are suffering from a hangover.
4. Wear a weight vest when training.
5. Wear an elevation training mask when working out on the double end bag.
6. Want to experience some real physical discomfort, try working out on the bag with a marble in your shoe.
7. To replicate unstable terrain, workout with sand, gravel or sawdust on the floor (be careful).
8. Practice hitting the bag with a light source beaming into your face.
9. Workout under poor lighting conditions.
10. Be creative, you are only limited by your imagination.

NOTES

Double End Bag Resources

Double End Bag Video

If you wish to explore additional information about double end bag training, I encourage you to check out the following video resource, available on amazon.com

- *Double End Bag Training*

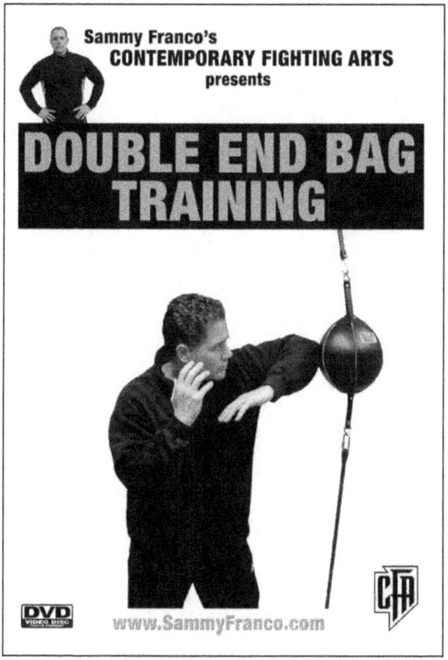

Double End Bag Training Video

Glossary

A

accuracy—The precise or exact projection of force. Accuracy is also defined as the ability to execute a combative movement with precision and exactness.

adaptability—The ability to physically and psychologically adjust to new or different conditions or circumstances of combat.

advanced first-strike tools—Offensive techniques that are specifically used when confronted with multiple opponents.

aerobic exercise—Literally, "with air." Exercise that elevates the heart rate to a training level for a prolonged period of time, usually 30 minutes.

affective preparedness – One of the three components of preparedness. Affective preparedness means being emotionally, philosophically, and spiritually prepared for the strains of combat. See cognitive preparedness and psychomotor preparedness.

aggression—Hostile and injurious behavior directed toward a person.

aggressive response—One of the three possible counters when assaulted by a grab, choke, or hold from a standing position. Aggressive response requires you to counter the enemy with destructive blows and strikes. See moderate response and passive response.

aggressive hand positioning—Placement of hands so as to imply aggressive or hostile intentions.

agility—An attribute of combat. One's ability to move his or her body quickly and gracefully.

amalgamation—A scientific process of uniting or merging.

ambidextrous—The ability to perform with equal facility on both the right and left sides of the body.

anabolic steroids - synthetic chemical compounds that resemble the male sex hormone testosterone. This performance-enhancing drug is known to increase lean muscle mass, strength, and endurance.

analysis and integration—One of the five elements of CFA's mental component. This is the painstaking process of breaking down various elements, concepts, sciences, and disciplines into their atomic parts, and then methodically and strategically analyzing, experimenting, and drastically modifying the information so that it fulfills three combative requirements: efficiency, effectiveness, and safety. Only then is it finally integrated into the CFA system.

anatomical striking targets—The various anatomical body targets that can be struck and which are especially vulnerable to potential harm. They include: the eyes, temple, nose, chin, back of neck, front of neck, solar plexus, ribs, groin, thighs, knees, shins, and instep.

anchoring - The strategic process of trapping the assailant's neck or limb in order to control the range of engagement during razing.

assailant—A person who threatens or attacks another person.

assault—The threat or willful attempt to inflict injury upon the person of another.

assault and battery—The unlawful touching of another person without justification.

assessment—The process of rapidly gathering, analyzing, and accurately evaluating information in terms of threat and danger. You can assess people, places, actions, and objects.

attack—Offensive action designed to physically control, injure, or kill another person.

attitude—One of the three factors that determine who wins a street fight. Attitude means being emotionally, philosophically, and spiritually liberated from societal and religious mores. See skills and knowledge.

attributes of combat—The physical, mental, and spiritual qualities that enhance combat skills and tactics.

awareness—Perception or knowledge of people, places, actions, and objects. (In CFA, there are three categories of tactical awareness: criminal awareness, situational awareness, and self-awareness.)

B

balance—One's ability to maintain equilibrium while stationary or moving.

blading the body—Strategically positioning your body at a 45-degree angle.

blitz and disengage—A style of sparring whereby a fighter moves into a range of combat, unleashes a strategic compound attack, and then quickly disengages to a safe distance. Of all sparring methodologies, the blitz and disengage most closely resembles a real street fight.

block—A defensive tool designed to intercept the assailant's attack by placing a non-vital target between the assailant's strike and your vital body target.

body composition—The ratio of fat to lean body tissue.

body language—Nonverbal communication through posture, gestures, and facial expressions.

body mechanics—Technically precise body movement during the execution of a body weapon, defensive technique, or other fighting maneuver.

body tackle – A tackle that occurs when your opponent haphazardly rushes forward and plows his body into yours.

body weapon—Also known as a tool, one of the various body parts that can be used to strike or otherwise injure or kill a criminal assailant.

burn out—A negative emotional state acquired by physically over- training. Some symptoms include: illness, boredom, anxiety, disinterest in training, and general sluggishness.

C

cadence—Coordinating tempo and rhythm to establish a timing pattern of movement.

cardiorespiratory conditioning—The component of physical fitness that deals with the heart, lungs, and circulatory system.

centerline—An imaginary vertical line that divides your body in half and which contains many of your vital anatomical targets.

choke holds—Holds that impair the flow of blood or oxygen to the brain.

circular movements—Movements that follow the direction of a curve.

close-quarter combat—One of the three ranges of knife and bludgeon combat. At this distance, you can strike, slash, or stab your assailant with a variety of close-quarter techniques.

cognitive development—One of the five elements of CFA's mental component. The process of developing and enhancing your fighting skills through specific mental exercises and techniques. See analysis and integration, killer instinct, philosophy, and strategic/tactical development.

cognitive exercises—Various mental exercises used to enhance fighting skills and tactics.

cognitive preparedness – One of the three components of preparedness. Cognitive preparedness means being equipped with the strategic concepts, principles, and general knowledge of combat. See affective preparedness and psychomotor preparedness.

combat-oriented training—Training that is specifically related to the harsh realities of both armed and unarmed combat. See ritual-oriented training and sport-oriented training.

combative arts—The various arts of war. See martial arts.

combative attributes—See attributes of combat.

combative fitness—A state characterized by cardiorespiratory and muscular/skeletal conditioning, as well as proper body composition.

combative mentality—Also known as the killer instinct, this is a combative state of mind necessary for fighting. See killer instinct.

combat ranges—The various ranges of unarmed combat.

combative utility—The quality of condition of being combatively useful.

combination(s)—See compound attack.

common peroneal nerve—A pressure point area located approximately four to six inches above the knee on the midline of the outside of the thigh.

composure—A combative attribute. Composure is a quiet and focused mind-set that enables you to acquire your combative agenda.

compound attack—One of the five conventional methods of attack. Two or more body weapons launched in strategic succession whereby the fighter overwhelms his assailant with a flurry of full speed, full-force blows.

conditioning training—A CFA training methodology requiring the practitioner to deliver a variety of offensive and defensive combinations for a 4-minute period. See proficiency training and street training.

contact evasion—Physically moving or manipulating your body to avoid being tackled by the adversary.

Contemporary Fighting Arts—A modern martial art and self-defense system made up of three parts: physical, mental, and spiritual.

conventional ground-fighting tools—Specific ground-fighting techniques designed to control, restrain, and temporarily incapacitate your adversary. Some conventional ground fighting tactics include: submission holds, locks, certain choking techniques, and specific striking techniques.

coordination—A physical attribute characterized by the ability to perform a technique or movement with efficiency, balance, and accuracy.

counterattack—Offensive action made to counter an assailant's initial attack.

courage—A combative attribute. The state of mind and spirit that enables a fighter to face danger and vicissitudes with confidence, resolution, and bravery.

creatine monohydrate—A tasteless and odorless white powder that mimics some of the effects of anabolic steroids. Creatine is a safe body-building product that can benefit anyone who wants to increase their strength, endurance, and lean muscle mass.

criminal awareness—One of the three categories of CFA awareness. It involves a general understanding and knowledge of the nature and dynamics of a criminal's motivations, mentalities, methods, and capabilities to perpetrate violent crime. See situational awareness and self-awareness.

criminal justice—The study of criminal law and the procedures associated with its enforcement.

criminology—The scientific study of crime and criminals.

cross-stepping—The process of crossing one foot in front of or behind the other when moving.

crushing tactics—Nuclear grappling-range techniques designed to crush the assailant's anatomical targets.

cue word - a unique word or personal statement that helps focus your attention on the execution of a skill, instead of its outcome.

D

deadly force—Weapons or techniques that may result in unconsciousness, permanent disfigurement, or death.

deception—A combative attribute. A stratagem whereby you delude your assailant.

decisiveness—A combative attribute. The ability to follow a tactical course of action that is unwavering and focused.

defense—The ability to strategically thwart an assailant's attack (armed or unarmed).

defensive flow—A progression of continuous defensive responses.

defensive mentality—A defensive mind-set.

defensive reaction time—The elapsed time between an assailant's physical attack and your defensive response to that attack. See offensive reaction time.

demeanor—A person's outward behavior. One of the essential factors to consider when assessing a threatening individual.

diet—A lifestyle of healthy eating.

disingenuous vocalization—The strategic and deceptive

utilization of words to successfully launch a preemptive strike at your adversary.

distancing—The ability to quickly understand spatial relationships and how they relate to combat.

distractionary tactics—Various verbal and physical tactics designed to distract your adversary.

double end bag—A small bag hung from the ceiling and anchored to the floor with two elastic cords. This unique training bag develops striking accuracy, speed, fighting rhythm, timing, eye-hand coordination, footwork and overall defensive skills.

double-leg takedown—A takedown that occurs when your opponent shoots for both of your legs to force you to the ground.

E

ectomorph—One of the three somatotypes. A body type characterized by a high degree of slenderness, angularity, and fragility. See endomorph and mesomorph.

effectiveness—One of the three criteria for a CFA body weapon, technique, tactic, or maneuver. It means the ability to produce a desired effect. See efficiency and safety.

efficiency—One of the three criteria for a CFA body weapon, technique, tactic, or maneuver. It means the ability to reach an objective quickly and economically. See effectiveness and safety.

emotionless—A combative attribute. Being temporarily devoid of human feeling.

endomorph—One of the three somatotypes. A body type characterized by a high degree of roundness, softness, and body fat. See ectomorph and mesomorph.

evasion—A defensive maneuver that allows you to strategically maneuver your body away from the assailant's strike.

evasive sidestepping—Evasive footwork where the practitioner moves to either the right or left side.

evasiveness—A combative attribute. The ability to avoid threat or danger.

excessive force—An amount of force that exceeds the need for a particular event and is unjustified in the eyes of the law.

experimentation—The painstaking process of testing a combative hypothesis or theory.

explosiveness—A combative attribute that is characterized by a sudden outburst of violent energy.

F

fear—A strong and unpleasant emotion caused by the anticipation or awareness of threat or danger. There are three stages of fear in order of intensity: fright, panic, and terror. See fright, panic, and terror.

feeder—A skilled technician who manipulates the focus mitts.

femoral nerve—A pressure point area located approximately 6 inches above the knee on the inside of the thigh.

fighting stance—Any one of the stances used in CFA's system. A strategic posture you can assume when face-to-face with an unarmed assailant(s). The fighting stance is generally used after you have launched your first-strike tool.

fight-or-flight syndrome—A response of the sympathetic nervous system to a fearful and threatening situation, during which it prepares your body to either fight or flee from the perceived danger.

finesse—A combative attribute. The ability to skillfully execute a movement or a series of movements with grace and refinement.

first strike—Proactive force used to interrupt the initial stages of an assault before it becomes a self-defense situation.

first-strike principle—A CFA principle that states that when physical danger is imminent and you have no other tactical option but to fight back, you should strike first, strike fast, and strike with authority and keep the pressure on.

first-strike stance—One of the stances used in CFA's system. A strategic posture used prior to initiating a first strike.

first-strike tools—Specific offensive tools designed to initiate a preemptive strike against your adversary.

fisted blows – Hand blows delivered with a clenched fist.

five tactical options – The five strategic responses you can make in a self-defense situation, listed in order of increasing level of resistance: comply, escape, de-escalate, assert, and fight back.

flexibility—The muscles' ability to move through maximum natural ranges. See muscular/skeletal conditioning.

focus mitts—Durable leather hand mitts used to develop and sharpen offensive and defensive skills.

footwork—Quick, economical steps performed on the balls of the feet while you are relaxed, alert, and balanced. Footwork is structured around four general movements: forward, backward, right, and left.

fractal tool—Offensive or defensive tools that can be used in more than one combat range.

fright—The first stage of fear; quick and sudden fear. See panic and terror.

full Beat – One of the four beat classifications in the Widow Maker Program. The full beat strike has a complete initiation and retraction phase.

G

going postal - a slang term referring to a person who suddenly and unexpectedly attacks you with an explosive and frenzied flurry of blows. Also known as postal attack.

grappling range—One of the three ranges of unarmed combat. Grappling range is the closest distance of unarmed combat from which you can employ a wide variety of close-quarter tools and techniques. The grappling range of unarmed combat is also divided into two planes: vertical (standing) and horizontal (ground fighting). See kicking range and punching range.

grappling-range tools—The various body tools and techniques that are employed in the grappling range of unarmed combat, including head butts; biting, tearing, clawing, crushing, and gouging tactics; foot stomps, horizontal, vertical, and diagonal elbow strikes, vertical and diagonal knee strikes, chokes, strangles, joint locks, and holds. See punching range tools and kicking range tools.

ground fighting—Also known as the horizontal grappling plane, this is fighting that takes place on the ground.

guard—Also known as the hand guard, this refers to a fighter's hand positioning.

guard position—Also known as leg guard or scissors hold, this is a ground-fighting position in which a fighter is on his back holding his opponent between his legs.

H

half beat – One of the four beat classifications in the Widow Maker Program. The half beat strike is delivered through the retraction phase of the proceeding strike.

hand positioning—See guard.

hand wraps—Long strips of cotton that are wrapped around the hands and wrists for greater protection.

haymaker—A wild and telegraphed swing of the arms executed by an unskilled fighter.

head-hunter—A fighter who primarily attacks the head.

heavy bag—A large cylindrical bag used to develop kicking, punching, or striking power.

high-line kick—One of the two different classifications of a kick. A kick that is directed to targets above an assailant's waist level. See low-line kick.

hip fusing—A full-contact drill that teaches a fighter to "stand his ground" and overcome the fear of exchanging blows with a stronger opponent. This exercise is performed by connecting two fighters with a 3-foot chain, forcing them to fight in the punching range of unarmed combat.

histrionics—The field of theatrics or acting.

hook kick—A circular kick that can be delivered in both kicking and punching ranges.

hook punch—A circular punch that can be delivered in both the punching and grappling ranges.

I

impact power—Destructive force generated by mass and velocity.

impact training—A training exercise that develops pain tolerance.

incapacitate—To disable an assailant by rendering him unconscious or damaging his bones, joints, or organs.

initiative—Making the first offensive move in combat.

inside position—The area between the opponent's arms, where he has the greatest amount of control.

intent—One of the essential factors to consider when assessing a threatening individual. The assailant's purpose or motive. See demeanor, positioning, range, and weapon capability.

intuition—The innate ability to know or sense something without the use of rational thought.

J

jersey Pull – Strategically pulling the assailant's shirt or jacket over his head as he disengages from the clinch position.

joint lock—A grappling-range technique that immobilizes the assailant's joint.

K

kick—A sudden, forceful strike with the foot.

kicking range—One of the three ranges of unarmed combat. Kicking range is the furthest distance of unarmed combat wherein you use your legs to strike an assailant. See grappling range and punching range.

kicking-range tools—The various body weapons employed in the kicking range of unarmed combat, including side kicks, push kicks, hook kicks, and vertical kicks.

killer instinct—A cold, primal mentality that surges to your consciousness and turns you into a vicious fighter.

kinesics—The study of nonlinguistic body movement communications. (For example, eye movement, shrugs, or facial gestures.)

kinesiology—The study of principles and mechanics of human movement.

kinesthetic perception—The ability to accurately feel your body during the execution of a particular movement.

knowledge—One of the three factors that determine who will win a street fight. Knowledge means knowing and understanding how to fight. See skills and attitude.

L

lead side -The side of the body that faces an assailant.

leg guard—See guard position.

linear movement—Movements that follow the path of a straight line.

low-maintenance tool—Offensive and defensive tools that require the least amount of training and practice to maintain proficiency. Low maintenance tools generally do not require preliminary stretching.

low-line kick—One of the two different classifications of a kick. A kick that is directed to targets below the assailant's waist level. (See high-line kick.)

lock—See joint lock.

M

maneuver—To manipulate into a strategically desired position.

MAP—An acronym that stands for moderate, aggressive, passive. MAP provides the practitioner with three possible responses to various grabs, chokes, and holds that occur from a standing position. See aggressive response, moderate response, and passive response.

Marathon des Sables (MdS) - a six-day, 156-mile ultramarathon held in southern Morocco, in the Sahara Desert. It is considered by many to be the toughest footrace on earth.

martial arts—The "arts of war."

masking—The process of concealing your true feelings from your opponent by manipulating and managing your body language.

mechanics—(See body mechanics.)

mental toughness - a performance mechanism utilizing a collection of mental attributes that allow a person to cope, perform and prevail through the stress of extreme adversity.

mental component—One of the three vital components of the CFA system. The mental component includes the cerebral aspects of fighting including the killer instinct, strategic and tactical development, analysis and integration, philosophy, and cognitive development. See physical component and spiritual component.

mesomorph—One of the three somatotypes. A body type classified by a high degree of muscularity and strength. The mesomorph possesses the ideal physique for unarmed combat. See ectomorph and endomorph.

mobility—A combative attribute. The ability to move your body quickly and freely while balanced. See footwork.

moderate response—One of the three possible counters when assaulted by a grab, choke, or hold from a standing position. Moderate response requires you to counter your opponent with a control and restraint (submission hold). See aggressive response and passive response.

modern martial art—A pragmatic combat art that has evolved to meet the demands and characteristics of the present time.

mounted position—A dominant ground-fighting position where a fighter straddles his opponent.

muscular endurance—The muscles' ability to perform the same

motion or task repeatedly for a prolonged period of time.

muscular flexibility—The muscles' ability to move through maximum natural ranges.

muscular strength—The maximum force that can be exerted by a particular muscle or muscle group against resistance.

muscular/skeletal conditioning—An element of physical fitness that entails muscular strength, endurance, and flexibility.

N

naked choke—A throat choke executed from the chest to back position. This secure choke is executed with two hands and it can be performed while standing, kneeling, and ground fighting with the opponent.

neck crush – A powerful pain compliance technique used when the adversary buries his head in your chest to avoid being razed.

neutralize—See incapacitate.

neutral zone—The distance outside the kicking range at which neither the practitioner nor the assailant can touch the other.

nonaggressive physiology—Strategic body language used prior to initiating a first strike.

nontelegraphic movement—Body mechanics or movements that do not inform an assailant of your intentions.

nuclear ground-fighting tools—Specific grappling range tools designed to inflict immediate and irreversible damage. Nuclear tools and tactics include biting tactics, tearing tactics, crushing tactics, continuous choking tactics, gouging techniques, raking tactics, and all striking techniques.

O

offense—The armed and unarmed means and methods of attacking a criminal assailant.

offensive flow—Continuous offensive movements (kicks, blows, and strikes) with unbroken continuity that ultimately neutralize or terminate the opponent. See compound attack.

offensive reaction time—The elapsed time between target selection and target impaction.

one-mindedness—A state of deep concentration wherein you are free from all distractions (internal and external).

ostrich defense—One of the biggest mistakes one can make when defending against an opponent. This is when the practitioner looks away from that which he fears (punches, kicks, and strikes). His mentality is, "If I can't see it, it can't hurt me."

P

pain tolerance—Your ability to physically and psychologically withstand pain.

panic—The second stage of fear; overpowering fear. See fright and terror.

parry—A defensive technique: a quick, forceful slap that redirects an assailant's linear attack. There are two types of parries: horizontal and vertical.

passive response—One of the three possible counters when assaulted by a grab, choke, or hold from a standing position. Passive response requires you to nullify the assault without injuring your adversary. See aggressive response and moderate response.

patience—A combative attribute. The ability to endure and tolerate difficulty.

perception—Interpretation of vital information acquired from your senses when faced with a potentially threatening situation.

philosophical resolution—The act of analyzing and answering various questions concerning the use of violence in defense of yourself and others.

philosophy—One of the five aspects of CFA's mental component. A deep state of introspection whereby you methodically resolve critical questions concerning the use of force in defense of yourself or others.

physical attributes—The numerous physical qualities that enhance your combative skills and abilities.

physical component—One of the three vital components of the CFA system. The physical component includes the physical aspects of fighting, such as physical fitness, weapon/technique mastery, and combative attributes. See mental component and spiritual component.

physical conditioning—See combative fitness.

physical fitness—See combative fitness.

positional asphyxia—The arrangement, placement, or positioning of your opponent's body in such a way as to interrupt your breathing and cause unconsciousness or possibly death.

positioning—The spatial relationship of the assailant to the assailed person in terms of target exposure, escape, angle of attack, and various other strategic considerations.

postal attack - see going postal.

power—A physical attribute of armed and unarmed combat. The amount of force you can generate when striking an anatomical target.

power generators—Specific points on your body that generate impact power. There are three anatomical power generators: shoulders, hips, and feet.

precision—See accuracy.

preemptive strike—See first strike.

premise—An axiom, concept, rule, or any other valid reason to modify or go beyond that which has been established.

preparedness—A state of being ready for combat. There are three components of preparedness: affective preparedness, cognitive preparedness, and psychomotor preparedness.

probable reaction dynamics - The opponent's anticipated or predicted movements or actions during both armed and unarmed combat.

proficiency training—A CFA training methodology requiring the practitioner to execute a specific body weapon, technique, maneuver, or tactic over and over for a prescribed number of repetitions. See conditioning training and street training.

proxemics—The study of the nature and effect of man's personal space.

proximity—The ability to maintain a strategically safe distance from a threatening individual.

pseudospeciation—A combative attribute. The tendency to assign subhuman and inferior qualities to a threatening assailant.

psychological conditioning—The process of conditioning the mind for the horrors and rigors of real combat.

psychomotor preparedness—One of the three components of preparedness. Psychomotor preparedness means possessing all of the physical skills and attributes necessary to defeat a formidable adversary. See affective preparedness and cognitive preparedness.

punch—A quick, forceful strike of the fists.

punching range—One of the three ranges of unarmed combat. Punching range is the mid range of unarmed combat from which the fighter uses his hands to strike his assailant. See kicking range and grappling range.

punching-range tools—The various body weapons that are employed in the punching range of unarmed combat, including finger jabs, palm-heel strikes, rear cross, knife-hand strikes, horizontal and shovel hooks, uppercuts, and hammer-fist strikes. See grappling-range tools and kicking-range tools.

Q

qualities of combat—See attributes of combat.

quarter beat - One of the four beat classifications of the Widow Maker Program. Quarter beat strikes never break contact with the assailant's face. Quarter beat strikes are primarily responsible for creating the psychological panic and trauma when Razing.

R

range—The spatial relationship between a fighter and a threatening assailant.

range deficiency—The inability to effectively fight and defend in all ranges of combat (armed and unarmed).

range manipulation—A combative attribute. The strategic manipulation of combat ranges.

range proficiency—A combative attribute. The ability to effectively fight and defend in all ranges of combat (armed and unarmed).

ranges of engagement—See combat ranges.

ranges of unarmed combat—The three distances (kicking range, punching range, and grappling range) a fighter might physically engage with an assailant while involved in unarmed combat.

raze – To level, demolish or obliterate.

razer – One who performs the Razing methodology.

razing – The second phase of the Widow Maker Program. A series of vicious close quarter techniques designed to physically and psychologically extirpate a criminal attacker.

razing amplifier - a technique, tactic or procedure that magnifies the destructiveness of your razing technique.

reaction dynamics—see probable reaction dynamics.

reaction time—The elapsed time between a stimulus and the response to that particular stimulus. See offensive reaction time and defensive reaction time.

rear cross—A straight punch delivered from the rear hand that crosses from right to left (if in a left stance) or left to right (if in a right stance).

rear side—The side of the body furthest from the assailant. See lead side.

reasonable force—That degree of force which is not excessive for a particular event and which is appropriate in protecting yourself or others.

refinement—The strategic and methodical process of improving or perfecting.

relocation principle—Also known as relocating, this is a street-fighting tactic that requires you to immediately move to a new location (usually by flanking your adversary) after delivering a compound attack.

repetition—Performing a single movement, exercise, strike, or action continuously for a specific period.

research—A scientific investigation or inquiry.

rhythm—Movements characterized by the natural ebb and flow of related elements.

ritual-oriented training—Formalized training that is conducted without intrinsic purpose. See combat-oriented training and sport-oriented training.

S

safety—One of the three criteria for a CFA body weapon, technique, maneuver, or tactic. It means that the tool, technique, maneuver or tactic provides the least amount of danger and risk for the practitioner. See efficiency and effectiveness.

scissors hold—See guard position.

scorching – Quickly and inconspicuously applying oleoresin capsicum (hot pepper extract) on your fingertips and then razing your adversary.

self-awareness—One of the three categories of CFA awareness. Knowing and understanding yourself. This includes aspects of yourself which may provoke criminal violence and which will promote a proper and strong reaction to an attack. See criminal awareness and situational awareness.

self-confidence—Having trust and faith in yourself.

self-enlightenment—The state of knowing your capabilities, limitations, character traits, feelings, general attributes, and motivations. See self-awareness.

set—A term used to describe a grouping of repetitions.

shadow fighting—A CFA training exercise used to develop and refine your tools, techniques, and attributes of armed and unarmed combat.

sharking – A counter attack technique that is used when your adversary grabs your razing hand.

shielding wedge - a defensive maneuver used to counter an unarmed postal attack.

situational awareness—One of the three categories of CFA awareness. A state of being totally alert to your immediate surroundings, including people, places, objects, and actions. (See criminal awareness and self-awareness.)

skeletal alignment—The proper alignment or arrangement of your body. Skeletal alignment maximizes the structural integrity of striking tools.

skills—One of the three factors that determine who will win a street fight. Skills refers to psychomotor proficiency with the tools and techniques of combat. See Attitude and Knowledge.

slipping—A defensive maneuver that permits you to avoid an assailant's linear blow without stepping out of range. Slipping can be accomplished by quickly snapping the head and upper torso sideways (right or left) to avoid the blow.

snap back—A defensive maneuver that permits you to avoid an assailant's linear and circular blows without stepping out of range. The snap back can be accomplished by quickly snapping the head backward to avoid the assailant's blow.

somatotypes—A method of classifying human body types or builds into three different categories: endomorph, mesomorph, and ectomorph. See endomorph, mesomorph, and ectomorph.

sparring—A training exercise where two or more fighters fight each other while wearing protective equipment.

speed—A physical attribute of armed and unarmed combat. The rate or a measure of the rapid rate of motion.

spiritual component—One of the three vital components of the CFA system. The spiritual component includes the metaphysical issues and aspects of existence. See physical component and mental component.

sport-oriented training—Training that is geared for competition and governed by a set of rules. See combat-oriented training and ritual-oriented training.

sprawling—A grappling technique used to counter a double- or single-leg takedown.

square off—To be face-to-face with a hostile or threatening assailant who is about to attack you.

stance—One of the many strategic postures you assume prior to or during armed or unarmed combat.

stick fighting—Fighting that takes place with either one or two sticks.

strategic positioning—Tactically positioning yourself to either escape, move behind a barrier, or use a makeshift weapon.

strategic/tactical development—One of the five elements of CFA's mental component.

strategy—A carefully planned method of achieving your goal of engaging an assailant under advantageous conditions.

street fight—A spontaneous and violent confrontation between two or more individuals wherein no rules apply.

street fighter—An unorthodox combatant who has no formal training. His combative skills and tactics are usually developed in the street by the process of trial and error.

street training—A CFA training methodology requiring the practitioner to deliver explosive compound attacks for 10 to 20 seconds. See condition ng training and proficiency training.

strength training—The process of developing muscular strength through systematic application of progressive resistance.

stress - physiological and psychological arousal caused by a stressor.

stressors - any activity, situation, circumstance, event, experience, or condition that causes a person to experience both physiological and psychological stress.

striking art—A combat art that relies predominantly on striking techniques to neutralize or terminate a criminal attacker.

striking shield—A rectangular shield constructed of foam and vinyl used to develop power in your kicks, punches, and strikes.

striking tool—A natural body weapon that impacts with the assailant's anatomical target.

strong side—The strongest and most coordinated side of your body.

structure—A definite and organized pattern.

style—The distinct manner in which a fighter executes or performs his combat skills.

stylistic integration—The purposeful and scientific collection of tools and techniques from various disciplines, which are strategically integrated and dramatically altered to meet three essential criteria: efficiency, effectiveness, and combative safety.

submission holds—Also known as control and restraint techniques, many of these locks and holds create sufficient pain to cause the adversary to submit.

system—The unification of principles, philosophies, rules, strategies, methodologies, tools, and techniques of a particular method of combat.

T

tactic—The skill of using the available means to achieve an end.

target awareness—A combative attribute that encompasses five strategic principles: target orientation, target recognition, target selection, target impaction, and target exploitation.

target exploitation—A combative attribute. The strategic maximization of your assailant's reaction dynamics during a fight. Target exploitation can be applied in both armed and unarmed encounters.

target impaction—The successful striking of the appropriate anatomical target.

target orientation—A combative attribute. Having a workable knowledge of the assailant's anatomical targets.

target recognition—The ability to immediately recognize appropriate anatomical targets during an emergency self-defense situation.

target selection—The process of mentally selecting the appropriate anatomical target for your self-defense situation. This is predicated on certain factors, including proper force response, assailant's positioning, and range.

target stare—A form of telegraphing in which you stare at the anatomical target you intend to strike.

target zones—The three areas in which an assailant's anatomical targets are located. (See zone one, zone two and zone three.)

technique—A systematic procedure by which a task is accomplished.

telegraphic cognizance—A combative attribute. The ability to recognize both verbal and non-verbal signs of aggression or assault.

telegraphing—Unintentionally making your intentions known to your adversary.

tempo—The speed or rate at which you speak.

terminate—To kill.

terror—The third stage of fear; defined as overpowering fear. See fright and panic.

timing—A physical and mental attribute of armed and unarmed combat. Your ability to execute a movement at the optimum moment.

tone—The overall quality or character of your voice.

tool—See body weapon.

traditional martial arts—Any martial art that fails to evolve and change to meet the demands and characteristics of its present environment.

traditional style/system—See traditional martial arts.

training drills—The various exercises and drills aimed at perfecting combat skills, attributes, and tactics.

trap and tuck – A counter move technique used when the adversary attempts to raze you during your quarter beat assault.

U

unified mind—A mind free and clear of distractions and focused on the combative situation.

use of force response—A combative attribute. Selecting the appropriate level of force for a particular emergency self-defense situation.

V

viciousness—A combative attribute. The propensity to be extremely violent and destructive often characterized by intense savagery.

violence—The intentional utilization of physical force to coerce, injure, cripple, or kill.

visualization—Also known as mental visualization or mental imagery. The purposeful formation of mental images and scenarios in the mind's eye.

W

warm-up—A series of mild exercises, stretches, and movements designed to prepare you for more intense exercise.

weak side—The weaker and more uncoordinated side of your body.

weapon and technique mastery—A component of CFA's physical component. The kinesthetic and psychomotor development of a weapon or combative technique.

weapon capability—An assailant's ability to use and attack with a particular weapon.

webbing - The first phase of the Widow Maker Program. Webbing is a two hand strike delivered to the assailant's chin. It is called Webbing because your hands resemble a large web that wraps around the enemy's face.

widow maker – One who makes widows by destroying husbands.

widow maker program – A CFA combat program specifically designed to teach the law abiding citizen how to use extreme force when faced with immediate threat of unlawful deadly criminal attack. The Widow Maker program is divided into two phases or methodologies: Webbing and Razing.

Y

yell—A loud and aggressive scream or shout used for various strategic reasons.

Z

zero beat – One of the four beat classifications of the Widow Maker, Feral Fighting and Savage Street Fighting Programs. Zero beat strikes are full pressure techniques applied to a specific target until it completely ruptures. They include gouging, crushing, biting, and choking techniques.

zone one—Anatomical targets related to your senses, including the eyes, temple, nose, chin, and back of neck.

zone three—Anatomical targets related to your mobility, including thighs, knees, shins, and instep.

zone two—Anatomical targets related to your breathing, including front of neck, solar plexus, ribs, and groin.

About Sammy Franco

With over 30 years of experience, Sammy Franco is one of the world's foremost authorities on armed and unarmed self-defense. Highly regarded as a leading innovator in combat sciences, Mr. Franco was one of the premier pioneers in the field of "reality-based" self-defense and combat instruction.

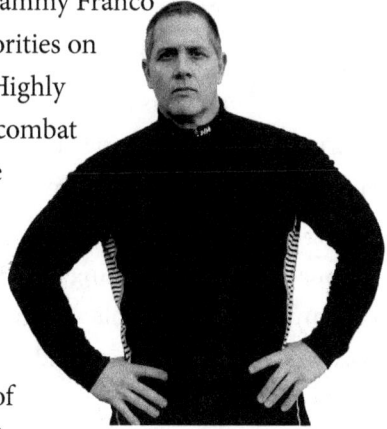

Sammy Franco is perhaps best known as the founder and creator of Contemporary Fighting Arts (CFA), a state-of-the-art offensive-based combat system that is specifically designed for real-world self-defense. CFA is a sophisticated and practical system of self-defense, designed specifically to provide efficient and effective methods to avoid, defuse, confront, and neutralize both armed and unarmed attackers.

Sammy Franco has frequently been featured in martial art magazines, newspapers, and appeared on numerous radio and television programs. Mr. Franco has also authored numerous books, magazine articles, and editorials and has developed a popular library of instructional videos.

Sammy Franco's experience and credibility in the combat science is unequaled. One of his many accomplishments in this field includes the fact that he has earned the ranking of a Law Enforcement Master Instructor, and has designed, implemented, and taught officer survival training to the United States Border Patrol (USBP). He has instructed members of the US Secret Service, Military Special Forces, Washington DC Police Department, Montgomery County, Maryland

Deputy Sheriffs, and the US Library of Congress Police. Sammy Franco is also a member of the prestigious International Law Enforcement Educators and Trainers Association (ILEETA) as well as the American Society of Law Enforcement Trainers (ASLET) and he is listed in the "Who's Who Director of Law Enforcement Instructors."

Sammy Franco is also a nationally certified Law Enforcement Instructor in the following curricula: PR-24 Side-Handle Baton, Police Arrest and Control Procedures, Police Personal Weapons Tactics, Police Power Handcuffing Methods, Police Oleoresin Capsicum Aerosol Training (OCAT), Police Weapon Retention and Disarming Methods, Police Edged Weapon Countermeasures and "Use of Force" Assessment and Response Methods.

Mr. Franco regularly conducts dynamic and enlightening seminars on different aspects of combat training, mental toughness and achieving personal peak performance.

On a personal level, Sammy Franco is an animal lover, who will go to great lengths to assist and rescue animals. Throughout the years, he's rescued everything from turkey vultures to goats. However, his most treasured moments are always spent with his beloved German Shepherd dogs.

For more information about Mr. Franco, you can visit his website at **SammyFranco.com** or follow him on Twitter **@RealSammyFranco**

Other Books by Sammy Franco

HEAVY BAG TRAINING

For Boxing, Mixed Martial Arts and Self-Defense
(Heavy Bag Training Series Book 1)

by Sammy Franco

The heavy bag is one of the oldest and most recognizable pieces of training equipment. It's used by boxers, mixed martial artists, self-defense practitioners, and fitness enthusiasts. Unfortunately, most people don't know how to use the heavy bag correctly. Heavy Bag Training teaches you everything you ever wanted to know about working out on the heavy bag. In this one-of-a-kind book, world-renowned self-defense expert Sammy Franco provides you with the knowledge, skills, and attitude necessary to maximize the training benefits of the bag. 8.5 x 5.5, paperback, photos, illus, 172 pages.

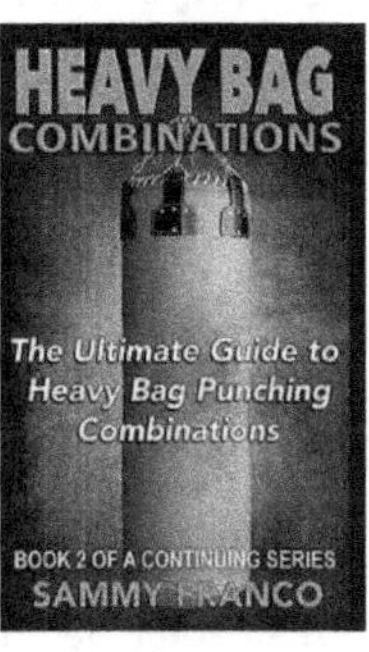

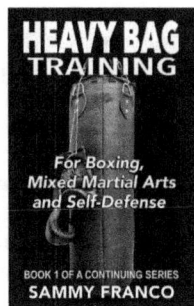

HEAVY BAG COMBINATIONS

The Ultimate Guide to Heavy Bag Punching Combinations
(Heavy Bag Training Series Book 2)

by Sammy Franco

Heavy Bag Combinations is the second book in Sammy Franco's best-selling Heavy Bag Training Series. This unique book is your ultimate guide to mastering devastating heavy bag punching combinations. With over 300+ photographs and detailed step-by-step instructions, Heavy Bag Combinations provides beginner, intermediate and advanced heavy bag workout combinations that will challenge you for the rest of your life! In fact, even the most experienced athlete will advance his fighting skills to the next level and beyond. 8.5 x 5.5, paperback, photos, illus, 248 pages.

THE COMPLETE BODY OPPONENT BAG BOOK

by Sammy Franco

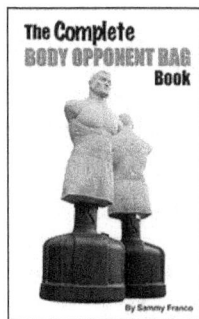

In this one-of-a-kind book, Sammy Franco teaches you the many hidden training features of the body opponent bag that will improve your fighting skills and boost your conditioning. With detailed photographs, step-by-step instructions, and dozens of unique workout routines, The Complete Body Opponent Bag Book is the authoritative resource for mastering this lifelike punching bag. It covers stances, punching, kicking, grappling techniques, mobility and footwork, targets, fighting ranges, training gear, time based workouts, punching and kicking combinations, weapons training, grappling drills, ground fighting, and dozens of workouts. 8.5 x 5.5, paperback, 139 photos, illustrations, 206 pages.

INVINCIBLE
Mental Toughness Techniques for Peak Performance

by Sammy Franco

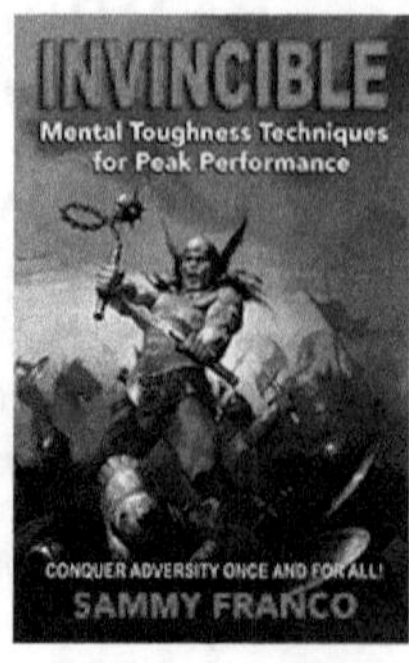

Invincible is a treasure trove of battle-tested techniques and strategies for improving mental toughness in all aspects of life. It teaches you how to unlock the true power of your mind and achieve success in sports, fitness, high-risk professions, self-defense, and other peak performance activities. However, you don't have to be an athlete or warrior to benefit from this unique mental toughness book. In fact, the mental skills featured in this indispensable program can be used by anyone who wants to reach their full potential in life. 8.5 x 5.5, paperback, photos, illus, 250 pages.

THE WIDOW MAKER PROGRAM
Extreme Self-Defense for Deadly Force Situations

by Sammy Franco

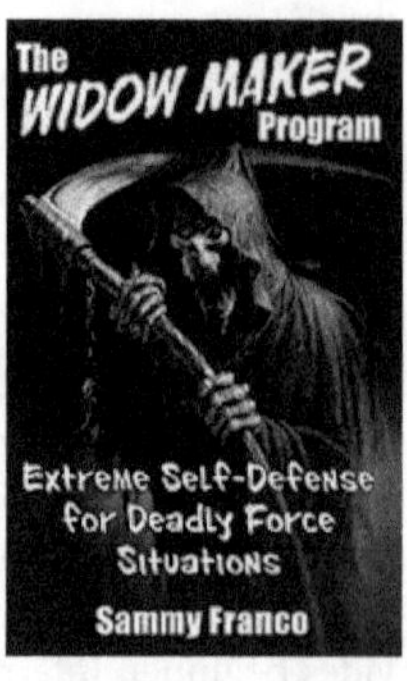

The Widow Maker Program is a shocking and revolutionary fighting style designed to unleash extreme force when faced with the immediate threat of an unlawful deadly criminal attack. In this unique book, self-defense innovator Sammy Franco teaches you his brutal and unorthodox combat style that is virtually indefensible and utterly devastating. With over 250 photographs and detailed step-by-step instructions, The Widow Maker Program teaches you Franco's surreptitious Webbing and Razing techniques. When combined, these two fighting methods create an unstoppable force capable of destroying the toughest adversary. 8.5 x 5.5, paperback, photos, illus, 218 pages.

FERAL FIGHTING
Advanced Widow Maker Fighting Techniques

by Sammy Franco

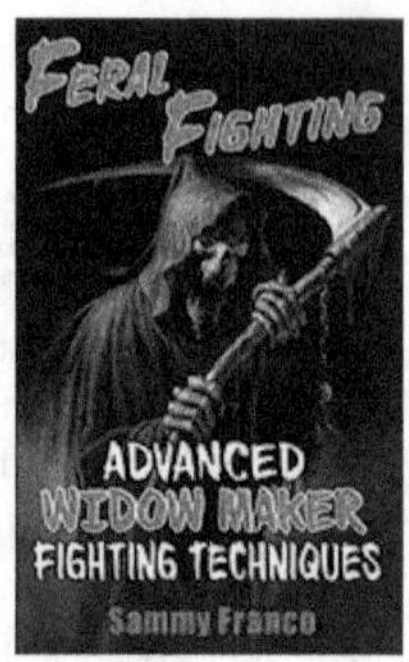

In this sequel, Sammy Franco marches forward with cutting-edge concepts and techniques that will take your self-defense skills to entirely new levels of combat performance. Feral Fighting includes Franco's revolutionary Shielding Wedge technique. When used correctly, it transforms you into an unstoppable human meat grinder, capable of destroying any criminal adversary. Feral Fighting also teaches you the cunning art or Scorching. Learn how to convert your fingertips into burning torches that generate over 2 million scoville heat units causing excruciating pain and temporarily blindness. 8.5 x 5.5, paperback, photos, illustrations, 204 pages.

MAXIMUM DAMAGE

Hidden Secrets Behind Brutal Fighting Combination

by Sammy Franco

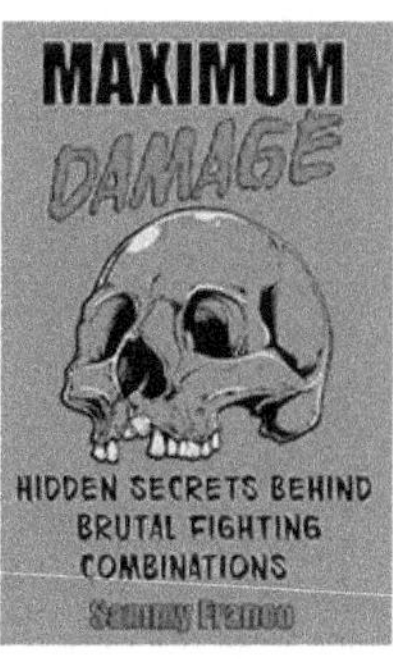

Maximum Damage teaches you the quickest ways to beat your opponent in the street by exploiting his physical and psychological reactions in a fight. Learn how to stay two steps ahead of your adversary by knowing exactly how he will react to your strikes before they are delivered. In this unique book, reality based self-defense expert Sammy Franco reveals his unique Probable Reaction Dynamic (PRD) fighting method. Probable reaction dynamics are both a scientific and comprehensive offensive strategy based on the positional theory of combat. Regardless of your style of fighting, PRD training will help you overpower your opponent by seamlessly integrating your strikes into brutal fighting combinations that are fast, ferocious and final! 8.5 x 5.5, paperback, 240 photos, illustrations, 238 pages.

SAVAGE STREET FIGHTING

Tactical Savagery as a Last Resort

by Sammy Franco

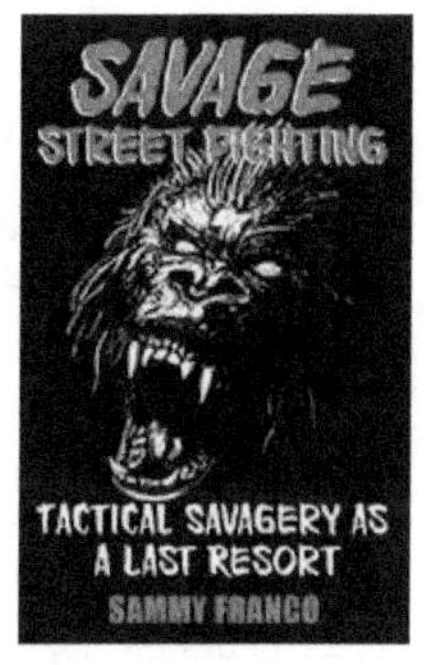

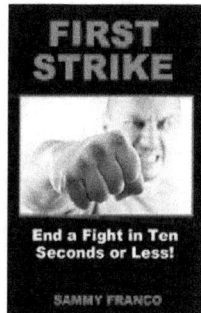

In this revolutionary book, Sammy Franco reveals the science behind his most primal street fighting method. Savage Street Fighting is a brutal self-defense system specifically designed to teach the law-abiding citizen how to use "Tactical Savagery" when faced with the immediate threat of an unlawful deadly criminal attack. Savage Street Fighting is systematically engineered to protect you when there are no other self-defense options left! With over 300 photographs and detailed step-by-step instructions, Savage Street Fighting is a must-have book for anyone concerned about real world self-defense. Now is the time to learn how to unleash your inner beast! 8.5 x 5.5, paperback, 317 photos, illustrations, 232 pages.

FIRST STRIKE

End a Fight in Ten Seconds or Less!

by Sammy Franco

Learn how to stop any attack before it starts by mastering the art of the preemptive strike. First Strike gives you an easy-to-learn yet highly effective self-defense game plan for handling violent close quarter combat encounters. First Strike will teach you instinctive, practical and realistic self-defense techniques that will drop any criminal attacker to the floor with one punishing blow. By reading this book and by practicing, you will learn the hard-hitting skills necessary to execute a punishing first strike and ultimately prevail in a self-defense situation. 8.5 x 5.5, paperback, photos, illustrations, 202 pages.

WAR MACHINE

How to Transform Yourself Into A Vicious & Deadly Street Fighter

by Sammy Franco

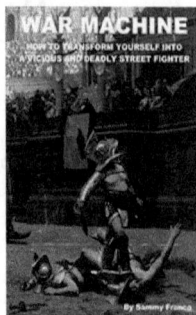

War Machine is a book that will change you for the rest of your life! When followed accordingly, War Machine will forge your mind, body and spirit into iron. Once armed with the mental and physical attributes of the War Machine, you will become a strong and confident warrior that can handle just about anything that life may throw your way. In essence, War Machine is a way of life. Powerful, intense, and hard. 11 x 8.5, paperback, photos, illustrations, 210 pages.

\KUBOTAN POWER

Quick and Simple Steps to Mastering the Kubotan Keychain

by Sammy Franco

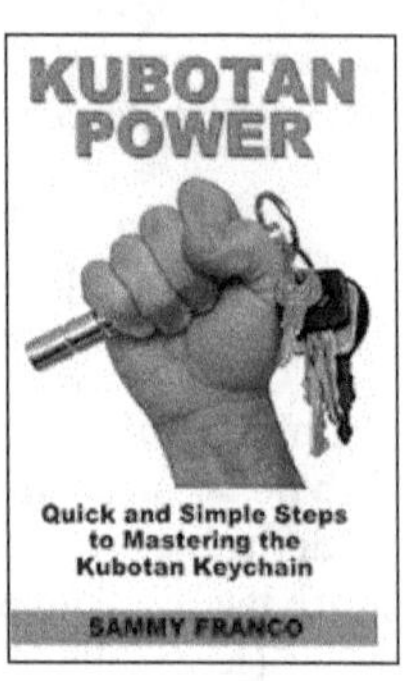

With over 290 photographs and step-by-step instructions, Kubotan Power is the authoritative resource for mastering this devastating self-defense weapon. In this one-of-a-kind book, world-renowned self-defense expert, Sammy Franco takes thirty years of real-world teaching experience and gives you quick, easy and practical kubotan techniques that can be used by civilians, law enforcement personnel, or military professionals. The Kubotan is an incredible self-defense weapon that has helped thousands of people effectively defend themselves. Men, women, law enforcement officers, military, and security professionals alike, appreciate this small and discreet self-defense tool. Unfortunately, however, very little has been written about the kubotan, leaving it shrouded in both mystery and ignorance. As a result, most people don't know how to unleash the full power of this unique personal defense weapon. 8.5 x 5.5, paperback, 290 photos, illustrations, 204 pages.

www.ingramcontent.com/pod-product-compliance
Lightning Source LLC
LaVergne TN
LVHW051624080426
835511LV00016B/2155